D1106178

The Park Avenue Face

"An honest look behind the curtain at today's advanced facial enhancement options from a world leader in the field and the one I trusted with my own face."

—Dr. Paul Nassif, plastic surgeon and television personality

"I have known Dr. Jacono for many years and have always been very impressed by his superior surgical skills, teaching abilities, and amazing results in facial rejuvenation. His surgical knowledge and teaching abilities have helped educate younger surgeons from all over the world, making Dr. Jacono an internationally renowned expert and one of New York City's premier facial plastic surgeons."

—Dr. Renato Saltz, internationally recognized plastic surgeon and past president of International Society of Aesthetic Plastic Surgery and the American Society for Aesthetic Plastic Surgery

"Dr. Jacono has been a go-to plastic surgery resource for over ten years. From commenting on celebrity procedures to discussing upcoming aesthetic trends, he's always on the pulse of what's hot."

—Beth Sobol, senior editor at E! News

"Social media are replete with information on facial rejuvenation. Though some of the information may be useful, more commonly it is self-serving and far from accurate. This work by an experienced professional accurately and effectively provides details of available options in a balanced fashion."

—Foad Nahai, MD, editor in chief of the *Aesthetic Surgery Journal* and past president of the American Society for Aesthetic Plastic Surgery and the International Society of Aesthetic Plastic Surgery

---

"The happiest patients are the ones who do their research and find the best fit for them. This book will help you understand what you want and how to get it—no matter where you live."

—Jamie Rosen, contributing editor at *Town & Country*

The Park Avenue Face

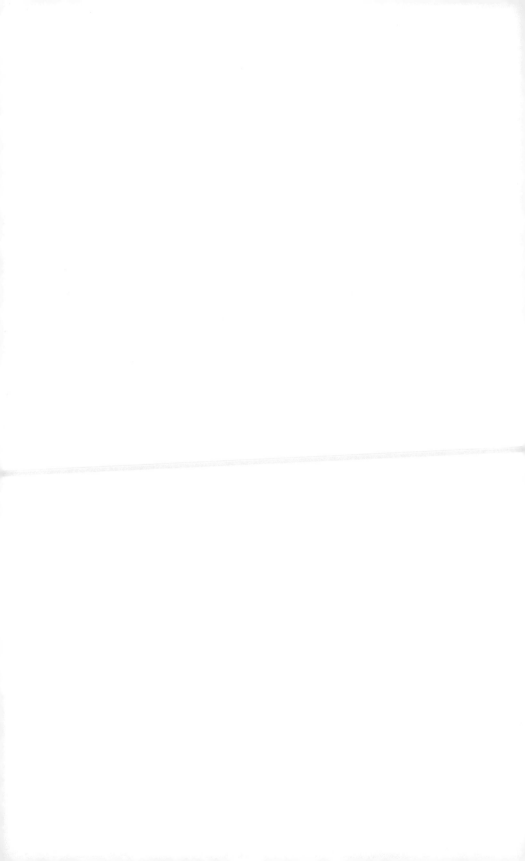

The Park Avenue Face

Secrets and Tips from a Top Facial Plastic Surgeon for
Flawless, Undetectable Procedures and Treatments

Andrew Jacono, MD, FACS

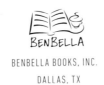

BENBELLA

BENBELLA BOOKS, INC.

DALLAS, TX

BenBella

BenBella Books, Inc.
10440 N. Central Expressway, Suite 800
Dallas, TX 75231
www.benbellabooks.com
Send feedback to feedback@benbellabooks.com

Printed in the United States of America
10 9 8 7 6 5 4 3 2 1

Library of Congress Cataloging-in-Publication Data
Names: Jacono, Andrew A., 1970- author.
Title: The Park Avenue face : secrets and tips from a top facial plastic
    surgeon for flawless, undetectable procedures and treatments / Andrew
    Jacono, MD, FACS.
Description: Dallas, TX : BenBella Books, Inc., [2019] | Includes
    bibliographical references and index.
Identifiers: LCCN 2018043942 (print) | LCCN 2018045558 (ebook) | ISBN
    9781948836234 (electronic) | ISBN 9781946885975 (trade cloth : alk. paper)
Subjects: LCSH: Face—Surgery—Popular works. | Surgery, Plastic—Popular
    works. | Skin—Care and hygiene—Popular works.
Classification: LCC RD523 (ebook) | LCC RD523 .J353 2019 (print) | DDC
    617.5/2059—dc23
LC record available at https://lccn.loc.gov/2018043942

Editing by Vy Tran
Copyediting by Elizabeth Degenhard
Proofreading by Lisa Story and Michael Fedison
Indexing by WordCo Indexing Services, Inc.
Text design by Faceout Studio, Paul Nielsen
Text composition by Aaron Edmiston
Author photo © William Hereford
Cover design by Emily Weigel
Cover photo © iStock / CoffeeAndMilk
Medical illustrations © William M. Winn
Printed by Versa Press

Distributed to the trade by Two Rivers Distribution, an Ingram brand
www.tworiversdistribution.com

Special discounts for bulk sales (minimum of 25 copies) are available. Please contact
bulkorders@benbellabooks.com.

I dedicate this book to my wonderful family.

To my children, Andrew, Arianna, Gavin, and Tallulah,
you infuse my life with such purpose, meaning, love, and fun.
I am so excited to watch you all pursue your dreams, and I
will be there by your side every step of the way.

To my partner, Jessica Wasmuth,
the love of my life, thank you for opening up new worlds to
me, for being my biggest cheerleader, and for understanding
my long hours and dedication to my craft.

CONTENTS

4 Begin with the Skin   71

5 Nonsurgical Facial Rejuvenation with Injectable Treatments   105

PART III   FINDING THE SURGICAL PROCEDURE THAT IS RIGHT FOR YOU

6 Open Your Eyes   131

7 Perfect Your Nose   159

8 Do Your Lips a Service   185

11 Don't Fear the Facelift   265

12 Anesthesia and Healing   297

INTRODUCTION

Welcome to the era of the face.

Never in human history have we been so obsessed with faces—our own faces, our family's faces, celebrity faces. Snapchat reveals to us a series of ephemeral faces; Instagram is an online album of faces experiencing the world; without "face," there is no Facebook. A face determines whether someone will swipe left or swipe right on a dating profile.

In fact, we should more accurately define this age as the era of the *digitally enhanced* face, when 33 percent of women and 20 percent of men admit to editing their dating profile photos with any of over 500 photo-editing apps.[1] Cell phone cameras are now designed for selfies, featuring high-tech portrait modes. We can flip through filters to soften harshness, mute redness, and create masterpiece selfies that show off our faces in their best (though not always most natural) light.

In many ways, the cell phone and the selfie have drastically changed how people think about their appearance. According to the American Academy of Facial Plastic and Reconstructive Surgery (AAFPRS), selfies and social media have also influenced those who are seeking facial enhancement.[2] Reports reveal a surge in millennial patients seeking minor to major treatments to the face, in many cases because they desire the trademark feature of a celebrity—Kylie Jenner's lips, for example—or because they want to prevent, rather than fix, an aging face. They ask for Botox, fillers, lip plumping procedures, and nose jobs. One in two plastic surgeons say they have seen an increase in procedures directly due to an increased facial awareness stemming from social media and the dissatisfaction that often comes with it.[3]

This is simply the state of the culture we live in right now, so you are not alone if you are secretly obsessing about your face. It is your central defining feature, and it influences how people perceive you at work, at play, at home. Fair or not, social media also influences how schools look at prospective students, how potential employers consider your application, and how likely potential clients are to hire you. They check media sites such as Facebook and LinkedIn for information about you—and they make snap judgments about your face.

But there is more to this cult of the face than meets the eye. As a dual board-certified facial plastic and reconstructive surgeon with a thriving practice in New York City, I specialize in and focus solely on faces. I have witnessed all these trends in my own clinics. I see all kinds of people in my office, for all kinds of reasons. I see young people concerned about the shape and size of their noses, the width and thickness of their lips, the contours of their cheeks. I see people aging in ways they don't like—people just approaching thirty, or forty, or fifty, who want to prevent or repair sagging skin, eye bags, jowls, and double chins. I also see teenagers and young professionals, people with injuries or facial irregularities that impede their lives, and classically beautiful people with complaints so minor that I couldn't have guessed what bothered them when they looked in the mirror. I see women of all ethnicities, from all different corners of the world, and, in much greater numbers than ever before, I see men. Fifteen years ago, I saw at most twelve men each year. Now I see at least a hundred.

I have also perceived a trend unique to the United States: a distinct difference between conceptions of beauty on the West Coast versus the East Coast. The difference between these two beauty ideals—and, more specifically, between the pictures people bring in, the celebrities they idealize, and the shapes of features they want from plastic surgeons—may not be so obvious to someone who is just beginning to consider some degree of facial enhancement, but I have learned to recognize it through a combination of cultural and aesthetic lenses. It is the difference between the demand for youthfulness that is driven by show business on the West Coast, and the demand for success that is driven by the workplace on the East Coast.

There is certainly no such thing as "the perfect look," and one style is not necessarily better than the other. However, it is likely that you relate to one ideal more than the other, and identifying the look that appeals to you is a necessary first step *before* you seek any degree of facial enhancement. Understanding the differences in these looks is a must, because the style of plastic surgery you desire should determine the techniques your surgeon will use, whether you think you want just a little Botox or a full-fledged facelift. The look you want should also influence your choice of plastic surgeon.

The United States is decades ahead of any other country in facial enhancement technology.[4] Noninvasive or minimally invasive techniques that stop short of actual surgery have become increasingly effective, and surgical procedures have also advanced to be simpler and less extreme, producing totally natural results. The best plastic surgeons and the most advanced devices are right here in the United States, and if you find an experienced and ethical plastic surgeon who understands and has been trained in the most recent techniques and procedures, you can fix what you don't like, restore what you've lost, or prevent what is coming to create a face you love. You will look rested. Refreshed. Younger. Never fake, never plastic.

Unfortunately, not every product, procedure, or technique will work for everyone. America may be the most advanced in facial enhancement, but it also has its share of scams—expensive "cosmeceuticals" that don't change your face any more than will a cheap moisturizer, devices and procedures that claim to be the next big thing but that don't give you results equivalent to the price you pay, and "quickie" surgical techniques that look fake or obvious. If you don't know what precisely you *do* want, what to ask, and what to expect, you could end up regretting you ever tried to change a thing about your face.

This is no reason to shy away from facial enhancement—it's why I've written this book! Knowledge is power, and this book will help you determine how you want to look and how to find the best medical professional. It will tell you everything you need to know about the most common procedures, from the least to the most invasive. Fortunately, getting the look you want is easier and safer than ever before—let this book be your guide.

How to Use This Book

This book will show you how to avoid the quacks, the fads, the financial waste, and the dangers that exist in the world of facial enhancement. It will tell you which procedures are worth the investment and which are a waste of your hard-earned cash. Typically, my patients have already spent thousands of dollars by the time they get to my office, and many of them still haven't gotten the results they expected. I want to help you avoid wasted time and money, so that you can get right to the techniques and procedures that will actually make the differences you are looking for. Some of them can transform your face, making you look years younger, or finally completely eliminating something that stands between you and the reflection you crave. From noninvasive treatments to minimally invasive procedures to more invasive surgeries, you will learn how to maximize your own beauty without wasting your money or wrecking your face.

In Part One, Choosing a Look for Your Lifestyle, I'll discuss the particulars of plastic surgery preferences in the United States, with distinct differences between the West Coast and East Coast styles. I'll also explain the importance of facial proportion for all ethnicities and discuss what to expect in each decade as your face and features gradually undergo changes. Aging is, of course, inevitable. As women grow older, the feminizing hormones estrogen and progesterone decrease, and more stereotypically male traits start to emerge in their faces. These traits can make a man look macho or handsome, but they tend to make a woman appear not only more masculine but angry and tired. Men are not immune to the effects of aging either. Their brows and upper eyelids droop and lower eyelid bags form, so they no longer look as rugged as they do downright exhausted. As the neck loosens, men appear not only older but heavier, even if they're in good shape.

In Part Two, Plastic Surgery 101: The Basics, you'll get a detailed primer of how to avoid becoming a plastic surgery victim. This section will teach you everything you need to know about finding the best plastic surgeon, how to identify red flags and potential scams, the questions you need to ask, and how to do the kind of research that will not only save you thousands of dollars but will help you get the results you want. It will break down the nuts and bolts of the least invasive procedures, like Botox, fillers, and peels, as well as give you detailed information about every aspect of what to expect when you have any kind of plastic surgery. From pre-surgery guidelines to post-op healing, from anesthesia to recovery, all of your questions will be answered.

In Part Three, Finding the Surgical Procedure That Is Right for You, I'll cover every area of the facial enhancement map, starting with skin care and moving from the brows and eyes down to ears, cheeks, noses, and lips to the chin, jawline, and neck. This section will include specific tips and guidance for men and for people of all ethnicities. You will see line drawings by veteran medical illustrator William Winn and before-and-after photographs that will give you an honest look at what good plastic surgery can accomplish: the wow factor.

The wow factor is at the heart of the work I do. It comes from my extensive experience as well as the passion and love I have for doing these procedures. I am very grateful for the gifts I've been given that allow me to match my technical expertise with an aesthetic sense that guides my work to produce a patient's desired results with minimal pain and stress. I adore my patients, who come to me from all over the world. They're incredibly interesting, engaged people who make me even more determined to be the best I can possibly be so they leave my office looking like themselves, only better. Over the course of my career, listening to patients describe their aesthetic goals and the realities of their jobs and lifestyles, I have developed techniques that respond specifically to their integrated needs and desires. The result is what I call the Park Avenue Face, a look that is defined by its naturalness, its realness.

That's the most important thing that you will learn in this book—the fact that facial enhancement procedures *can* look natural. They *can* fix something that has bothered you for years or restore a more youthful appearance if aging has created facial imbalance. This truth is at the heart of the Park Avenue Face, defining the look as well as this guide. The Park Avenue Face is about enhancing your beauty while maintaining your identity. You *can* have a simple procedure that will improve the basic balance and harmony of your facial features.

Thanks to modern surgical techniques, plastic surgery is safe and straightforward when performed by an experienced and ethical physician. And it should give you results that are anything but plastic. By the end of this book, you'll know exactly what procedure will really work for you, and you'll also know whether you are ready and willing to take action, whether you want to get a simple injection or a full-on facelift. You'll be fully prepared.

Most importantly, this book will tell you what you need to know to make sure your results look natural. The only way anyone will know you had plastic surgery is if you decide to tell them. I know that you want people to see *you* rather than what you perceive to be your flaws, but I also know you don't want to show up in public with a face that makes people whisper, "Have they had work done?" A natural look is the single most important component of the Park Avenue Face. In other words, I don't want you to be self-conscious due to your flaws or due to the fixes. I want you to be *fabulous*.

Since we live in the era of the face, I want *your* face to reflect the person you have always been and the person you strive to be, not a cartoon or a caricature or someone you don't recognize in the mirror. If you have a feature that bothers you, such as a nose bump or thin lips, or if you are disturbed by the way aging has made your eyes droop or your neck crease, or if you are self-conscious about a weak chin, bags under your eyes, or jawline droop, whether for personal, social, or professional reasons (or all of them), plastic surgery can help you achieve a more youthful face that looks like you, filtered and enhanced to fully express your beautiful personality. Because, in the end, the Park Avenue Face is about *individuality* as much as it is about *beauty*. They are two sides of the same coin, and the most knowledgeable doctors and aestheticians understand the importance of equally emphasizing these two priorities for facial enhancement.

Last, but certainly not least, Park Avenue doesn't have a monopoly on natural beauty. There are beautiful people on every avenue in the city, and in every other city, state, and country. But Park Avenue can be the bar to which you hold your plastic surgeon. Because your face is important. It is uniquely yours, the logo for your personal brand. It is what attracts others to you—or doesn't. It is the part of you that "interfaces" with the world, and if it doesn't feel right to you, if there is something on your face or about your face that makes you want to hide, it can be very difficult to feel comfortable, let alone confident, in your virtual or actual social interactions.

So read on. You *can* have the Park Avenue face, no matter who you are and where you live. Everything beautiful about you can be written on your face—and that, in my world, is perfection.

---

1 "Surprise! Many Men and Women Retouch Their Dating Profile Photos," *Meitu*, June 9, 2016, https://corp.meitu.com/en/news/news/21.html.

2 "Social Media Makes Lasting Impact on Industry—Becomes Cultural Force, Not Fad," American Academy of Facial Plastic and Reconstructive Surgery, January 29, 2018, https://www.aafprs.org/media/stats_polls/m_stats.html.

3 Ibid.

4 "Demand for Cosmetic Surgery Procedures Around the World Continues to Skyrocket—USA, Brazil, Japan, Italy and Mexico Ranked in the Top Five Countries," International Society of Aesthetic Plastic Surgery, June 27, 2017, https://www.isaps.org/wp-content/uploads/2017/10/GlobalStatistics.PressRelease2016-1.pdf.

PART
I

CHOOSING
A LOOK
FOR YOUR LIFESTYLE

1

East Coast Versus West Coast

What's Your Beauty Style?

What makes a person beautiful?

Beauty is hard to define or even describe. When you see a beautiful person, you're not always able to explain what it is that makes him or her beautiful. You just know; it's a feeling, an emotional response. It's not always as simple as a single feature or a combination of features. This is why one person might look at da Vinci's famous painting of the Mona Lisa and find her ravishing, and someone else might find her smile odd, her lack of eyebrows unsettling. I believe nothing holds more truth than the old adage *Beauty is in the eye of the beholder.*

Beauty is also defined by cultural norms. What Caucasians find beautiful is not necessarily what Asians or African Americans or Latinos find beautiful. For example, when I am consulting with an African American or Asian patient for a rhinoplasty, they want to maintain the ethnic character of their nose—a wider nasal bridge and nasal tip, not a narrow nose with an elevated tip that many of my female Caucasian patients request.

You can break these aesthetic differences down even further: What the French find beautiful might differ from what the Koreans, the Italians, the Americans, the Kenyans, or the Brazilians find beautiful. But every culture can agree that, no matter the specific arrangement of your features, your face is your personal signature.

What Patients Want

I see patients of every age, ethnicity, and gender in my office, all of whom have different needs, concerns, and desires. However, every single one of them falls into one of these four categories:

1. They want to preserve their features.
2. They want to restore what has aged.
3. They want to balance what is imbalanced, such as a crooked nose or droopy eyelids.
4. They want to refine what they perceive to be deficient or excessive, such as lips that are too thin or an overly long chin.

For example, many of my younger patients want to fix their noses or plump their lips. Those who are in their early thirties want to protect themselves from signs of aging, often with a more aggressive skin-care regimen. Many of my patients who are in their forties and fifties want to restore features that have changed with age, such as their eyes, cheeks, jawline, neck, or skin.

In all my experience, I have identified two very different ways that patients tend to approach facial procedures and rejuvenation: the West Coast style, which I believe is driven by the current Hollywood aesthetic, with its preference for youthfulness; and the East Coast style, which is my personal aesthetic and the foundation of the Park Avenue Face.

The West Coast style is about *changing* your personal signature.

The East Coast style is about *maintaining* your personal signature.

Neither style is right or wrong. Your aesthetic is unique to you. You might like certain aspects of the West Coast style, such as amplified lips, and other aspects of the East Coast style, such as subtle changes to your eyes. You might identify with the defining philosophies and results of one sole style. Your personal opinions and desires should guide your decision-making when it comes to plastic surgery; it is important that you do not allow your plastic surgeon to force you into their style rather than respect yours. If it makes you happy, ask for it. I do think it is important to clarify that just because a surgeon practices on the East or West Coast does not mean he or she subscribes to either of these styles. In Chapter 3, I will discuss how to figure out if a plastic surgeon you are considering is the right fit for your personal style.

The West Coast Style

The West Coast style is big, bold, brazen. Most significantly, it's about the cult of youth.

A West Coast–style face is hard to miss—and that's the point! Features are overtly sexualized: big, puffy lips; smooth, rounded cheeks; pinched, turned-up noses; frozen foreheads; distinctively arched brows; wide-open eyes. Looking like you've had work done is even a point of pride for many devotees of the West Coast style. I realized this recently when I attended a charity event in Beverly Hills. As I gazed around the room, I realized that all the women there between the ages of thirty-five and sixty looked related. Literally every single one of them had beautifully highlighted blonde hair and the same shapely thin nose, large lips, smooth cheeks and foreheads, and tight jawlines.

Some of the West Coast aesthetic is driven by patients and some of it is doctor preference, but most of all, it's what's in the public's mind when people think of plastic surgery, because the West Coast style is driven by Hollywood. The Hollywood stars who we see on the big screen, the television screen, or the computer screen often look like they have had work done and appear unnaturally young.

Is this their fault? I don't think so. This puts Hollywood stars (and aspirants) in an almost impossible position. Their lives and their appearance are hyper-exposed. Ever since high-definition video became the norm, we are able to see every pore and wrinkle on their faces. So when women tell their doctors or surgeons that they want rounder, younger-looking faces, it might be because they like the look—or it might more likely be because the entertainment industry *demands* it. Dramatic, age-reversing plastic surgery is so prevalent that Oscar-winner Frances McDormand, who has never "mutated [herself] in any way,"[1] is seen as an anomaly among her peers. Born in 1957, McDormand is aging in a perfectly normal, lovely way, yet almost every other working actress her age has a much smoother, rounded, and wrinkle-free face. These performers *need* to look young for as long as possible, and they know that pouty lips and unlined faces are what get them cast. And so the West Coast style endures. By logical extension, it's fair to conclude that the West Coast style is partially driven by the desire for fame. For most aspiring stars, ascension up the ladder of fame requires conforming to the physical characteristics of their industry's dominant archetype.

These show business stars or wannabe stars know that their image and their brand are one and the same. Whether you're launching a career as an actress or an aspiring social media influencer or YouTube vlogger, your image is one of the most important aspects of your business plan, because your image *is* your brand. Those whose looks are considered more plain and unremarkable are less likely to succeed. All brand marketing also works the same way. That's why when you look at any magazine or advertisement, you'll see many perfect bodies and perfect faces—the freckles, wrinkles, blemishes, and cellulite were left on the cutting room floor.

Is this fair? No. Is it realistic? No. Especially considering the astonishing double standard these practices reinforce. A man can age "gracefully" and be cast as the hero into his fifties and sixties, while his love interest is considered a dinosaur should she dare to approach forty. Ageism in Hollywood is most definitely not a new trend, but with the advent of noninvasive and surgical techniques, as well as injectables such as fillers and Botox, the cult of youth has invaded the offices of medical practitioners—and not always with the best results.

In this age of social media and the internet, there is no place where this phenomenon is more apparent than the universe of Instagram influencers. Most of the top beauty Instagrammers look like Barbie dolls, with their enhanced breasts showcased in revealing tank tops and their inflated lips even more exaggerated with on-trend makeup and techniques, like contouring and lip kits. Their looks have earned them millions of followers. Other beauty bloggers who are attractive and knowledgeable but have an understated appearance may struggle with attracting more than 500 followers. If you're trying to be famous at this point in time in America, you must either succumb to the current archetype or find some other way to showcase your talent in a truly unique way, which is extremely difficult to do.

It's impossible not to notice how the fashion, beauty, and celebrity media are showcasing younger and younger stars. A generation or so ago, during the 1990s era of the supermodel, models such as Christy Turlington, Naomi Campbell, and Cindy Crawford were in their twenties, working into their thirties. They weren't a size zero. They weren't Botoxed and filled. They looked their age, and we looked at them because they were uniquely beautiful.

Why are the cover girls of today so young? Because this is what sells. The West Coast style is always going to aim for a look that is as young as possible, creating features that are molded to the current celebrity archetype.

This becomes a problem for young women who are still figuring themselves out, growing into their features, but who feel pressured to conform to the West Coast style. These women might already be very attractive, but they become convinced that they need a lot of injectables as well as surgery to compete with everyone else whose looks follow the West Coast trends. Even if they don't have a big nose, they'll get the smallest, thinnest nose possible. Even if they already have wonderfully shaped or distinctive lips, they'll get them plumped up to have the biggest lips possible. They often use Kylie Jenner as a role model. Those who prefer more subtle enhancements often say that Jenner has completely altered her face and is unrecognizable, while many who prefer the brazen West Coast style argue that she's made herself look better—and take a photo of her to their surgeon and ask for the same nose and lips.

I think this is one of the reasons why so many television, movie, and music stars end up on botched plastic surgery websites, with their faces altered beyond recognition. It's doubly hard for them, because their faces are their brand, and there is no shortage of reminders of what they once looked like when they were younger. Comparisons are easy to make, and so are snarky comments. This is why one of the most common statements I hear is, "If celebrities who have all the money in the world, and the access to the best doctors, end up looking obviously fake and plastic, what chance do I have at looking good but still like myself after surgery?"

When prospective patients who prefer the West Coast style come to see me, they usually request very specific changes. They pull out photos and tell me that they want to look exactly like someone who is overly Photoshopped or obviously filtered on Instagram. They're looking for a level of perfection that is unrealistic and usually unattainable—because these photos aren't real. Even though they know deep down that these images are altered, there's still a disconnect. They don't care that the person they want to emulate is fake. They're convinced that this is what they want.

In fact, I've had people fly in from all over the world who are already drop-dead gorgeous yet want *more* work done. Most of them have had multiple procedures, and they already look amazing. I believe that some patients will look better if they leave their faces alone. Unless you've been botched, no one needs a facelift every two years! More is not always more.

What concerns me is when the West Coast style is used to significantly change a person's features to meet the standards of show business but in a way that isn't necessarily best for their face. Undergoing invasive or noninvasive procedures might work in the short term, but feeling forced to go in that direction in the hopes of becoming famous can be distressing in the long run—you lose your personal identity. I don't think that the average consumer of plastic surgery, whatever style they prefer, wants to do that at all. I don't think beauty is worth the cost of losing what makes your face uniquely yours.

Plastic Surgery Is Increasingly Popular with Men

With the American male grooming market now worth $3.5 billion, men are clearly feeling the need to look youthful well into their forties, fifties, and sixties. Statistics from the American Society for Aesthetic Plastic Surgery show that surgery is becoming increasingly popular with men as a way to deal with image maintenance.[2] Though women are still more commonly judged by their appearance, men are aware that in a hyper-competitive, ageist job market, facial plastic surgery is a tool they can use to look confident, youthful, and energetic, which may help them get ahead.

The overwhelming majority of men who come to me prefer the East Coast style. They want to look like themselves, just

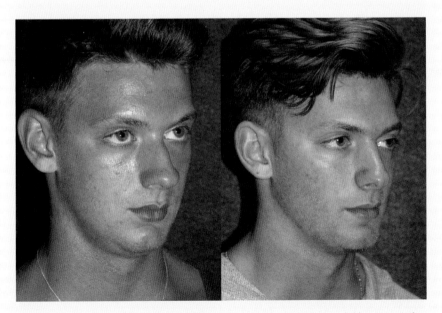

Figure 1: Before (left) and after (right) of a man who underwent a rhinoplasty and chin augmentation to harmonize his facial balance. Reducing the size of his nose and increasing the size of his chin creates a more masculine appearance. Surgery for men should not be overdone, to avoid feminizing the face.

refreshed and rejuvenated. The most common surgeries I perform on men are rhinoplasty, hair transplant, blepharoplasty
(eyelid lift), neck lift, and facelift. When surgery is skillfully
done, it's hard to detect (Figure 1).

Let me reiterate, however, that this will always be a matter of
personal choice, as there is no right or wrong look. Those who
love the West Coast style should go for it! It's only wrong when
you ask a surgeon for one style and he or she gives you another.

The East Coast Style

Where the West Coast style idolizes youth, the East Coast
style idolizes professional success. In New York—particularly
on Park Avenue—age equals wisdom, experience, respect, and
power. Obvious and distracting signs of aging, such as sagging
necks, wrinkled cheeks, pouched eyes, and droopy jowls are
just as undesirable on the East Coast as they are anywhere
else, but on Park Avenue, the fear is that these outer traits
will negatively impact how one projects his or her inner traits:
ambition, talent, and ability. This shouldn't be the case, of
course—wrinkles *shouldn't* disqualify anyone from advance-
ment or esteem. But the truth is that they might. Then again,
an obviously fake, surgically enhanced face is also likely to
make a bad impression.

Overall, I find that my typical patients don't want to look
like they have had any work done. They want to fight the signs

of aging, but, just as importantly, they want to maintain the features that make their faces unique. They want a face that aligns with their ethnicity, a face that makes them feel competitive in their careers, and, most of all, a face that looks *natural*. They want to look like themselves. They want to re-create their personal signature, not change it. The last thing they want is for people to notice a feature that artificially stands out, even if it was beautifully done.

I should add that the Park Avenue Face patient rarely lives on Park Avenue (though my office and surgical suite are located there). In fact, my patients come to me from all over the world. They know the old saying, "Plastic surgery should whisper, not scream"—and this defines their aesthetic. They want a natural outcome and are very apprehensive about looking different in any obvious way.

I love being able to provide my patients with natural-looking, individualized results. This is what my patients ask for. They've done their due diligence and interviewed other surgeons (a process you'll learn about in Chapter 3). They've looked at hundreds of before-and-after photos. They have a firm idea of what they want and have chosen me because my aesthetic is evident.

I don't think my patients are imbued with the "less is more" philosophy—they simply look amazingly *wow*. They aren't underdone; my work is unobtrusive. Many people assume that if you want to look natural after surgery, you can't have too much done, but this is not true. Natural results are possible even with invasive plastic surgical procedures when they are

Changing One Feature on Your Face Will Let Your Personal Identity Shine

An issue that transcends the East Coast versus West Coast style is when someone has a distorting facial feature that throws off the entire aesthetic balance of his or her face. This is where plastic surgery can be a tremendous help, especially for anyone who has ears that stick out or a really small chin or their grandfather's distinctive and enormously hooked nose. When a singular feature is significantly distracting, it can take away from a person's facial identity. In other words, if you have beautiful facial structure—gorgeous eyes, nice cheekbones, a shapely forehead and brows—but a disproportionately misshapen nose, the eye will naturally be drawn *only* to that nose, and it can literally make those other features invisible.

A guiding principle for evaluating this is the rule of thirds originally described by Leonardo da Vinci. The facial thirds extend from the hairline to the glabella line (eyebrows), the brow to the base of the nose, and the base of the nose to the chin. In a well-proportioned and attractive face, the resulting thirds are equal (Figure 2).

Take a good look at these before-and-after photos, because this is a wonderful example of how one surgical procedure can completely transform the thirds of the face (Figure 3).

Before her surgery, this woman's face looked long, narrow, and tired. The length of her nose made her middle third appear too long, overemphasizing her chin and jawline and making her cheekbones look smaller and flatter. The width and droopiness of her nasal tip dragged the appearance of her brows and

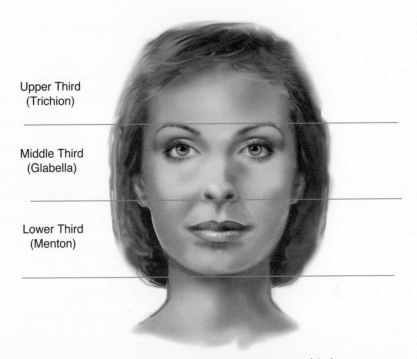

Upper Third
(Trichion)

Middle Third
(Glabella)

Lower Third
(Menton)

Figure 2: Leonardo da Vinci's rule of thirds describes three separate areas of the face.

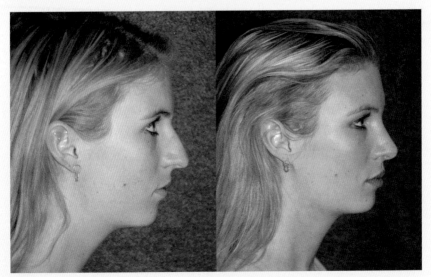

Figure 3: Before (left) and after (right) of a young woman who underwent a rhinoplasty (nose job). Her old nose had created an aesthetic disproportion, which affected every other feature on her face. After surgery, her cheekbones, lips, and eyes look improved without having had any surgery.

eyes downward, making them look tired. Her personal identity was hidden by one feature: her nose.

All I did for her was a rhinoplasty, which shortened the nose and lifted and defined the nasal tip. Afterward, you can easily see how this patient's cheekbones look fuller and higher and the middle of her face looks thinner, even though her weight hasn't changed. Her chin looks smaller. Her eyes look more open and her brows look more arched. Her lips are in better proportion. That's because her old nose had created an aesthetic disproportion, which affected every other feature on her face. I love how one small change can have an enormous effect on someone's appearance. She still looks like herself—only better.

This is why, as you'll learn in Chapter 3, it is always better to start slow. This patient didn't need anything else done to her face, even though other surgeons she'd consulted insisted that she did. They told her she needed a brow lift, fat put into her cheeks, her chin reduced, and work on her lips. If she'd had all of that additional work on top of the rhinoplasty, she *would* have looked distorted—her cheeks would have been too big and rounded, her brows too high, her chin too small, and her lips gargantuan. She would have come to me in tears, asking me to reverse her brow lift, suck the fat out of her cheeks, give her a chin implant, and dissolve the filler in her lips.

You can always do more should you want to—but only when *you* want to, not when a doctor tells you it's a must!

performed with balance and respect for facial tissues. A light touch is required. Their results leave them with the proper proportions, which I'll discuss in the next chapter, that make them look refreshed and younger—yet still completely themselves.

------

1 Frank Bruni, "A Star Who Has No Time for Vanity," *New York Times*, October 15, 2014, https://www.nytimes.com/2014/10/19/arts/frances-mcdormand-true-to-herself-in-hbos-olive-kitteridge.html.

2 "Cosmetic Surgery National Data Bank Statistics 2012," The American Society for Aesthetic Plastic Surgery, 2012, https://www.surgery.org/sites/default/files/ASAPS-2012-Stats.pdf.

2 It's All About Proportion

Angelina Jolie is widely considered to have one of the most recognizable and beautiful faces in the world. So is Nefertiti, the Egyptian queen. Gorgeous faces like theirs arouse our senses in a way that is more visceral than it is intellectual. They speak to us without saying a word.

What are the essential characteristics of a beautiful face? As I wrote in Chapter 1, beauty is, of course, subjective, and different cultures have different beauty standards. But the answer to this question is crucial, especially if a plastic surgeon is going to modify facial features with the intention of rejuvenating a patient's face and making it appear more attractive. As a surgeon, my goal is not to make everyone look the same but to better define the science of beauty so that I can best unlock the potential that exists in every person's face.

So how can you use the highly idiosyncratic notions of beauty to help you get the plastic surgery results you want? By understanding *proportion*.

Proportion Defines Beauty

Beauty makes us feel good. We can't explain it, but when we see it, we just *know* it. Whether conveyed through an amazing work of art or an amazing house or an amazing face, beauty stands the test of time.

Beauty trends—specific features, elements of an overarching aesthetic—come and go, but the essence of beauty is unchanging. And our ability to recognize beauty is rooted in our very human nature. It's simple: We're programmed to respond to proportion.

In one study, British researchers asked white, Asian, and Latino participants from a dozen European countries to select attractive faces from a diverse collection, and they all chose the same ones.[1] Even babies have a sense of what is attractive, as other studies have shown that infants as young as three to six months gaze longer at conventionally nice-looking faces than others that are considered plain.[2] These babies have no idea what social norms of beauty are; they're instinctively reacting to balanced facial proportions.

My goal is to give patients the best possible proportions to result in the high standards of the Park Avenue Face. For example, beauties such as Nefertiti, Angelina Jolie, and Audrey Hepburn have a very defined and elegant posterior aspect to their jawlines. The average patient wouldn't know to use that kind of technical description, but they do know that the shape of Nefertiti's, Angelina's, and Audrey's chins and jawlines make their faces attractive and distinctive.

I create balance for my patients by respecting and enhancing the natural proportion that exists everywhere in nature; this proportion is referred to as the golden ratio. When one's face reflects the golden ratio, it looks beautiful, natural, and rejuvenated. When it doesn't, it looks altered, imbalanced, and distorted. The proportions are off. You can't stop staring at it, either—for all the wrong reasons.

Using the Golden Ratio to Get the Proportions You Want

Have you ever been to a Gothic cathedral in France or the Cloisters Museum in Manhattan? If so, you've seen exquisite examples of medieval art. But what you didn't see was an accurate representation of the human body and the human face—the techniques available to artists during that period were limited, meaning images remained flat and one-dimensional. With the Renaissance, however, proportion and perspective entered the picture (literally!), and images in art became as realistic as they had been during the classical period, when ancient Greeks and Romans perfected figurative sculpture. Faces like those of Botticelli's Venus or Raphael's Sistine Madonna are as transporting now as they were when they were painted in the fifteenth and sixteenth centuries. Why? Because the artists used what is called the divine proportion, or the golden mean—what is commonly referred to now as the golden ratio.

The golden ratio is a term for the mathematical ratio of 1:1.618 and describes the relationship of one length to another. It is represented by the Greek letter φ, or *phi*, named for the acclaimed Greek sculptor Phidias who regularly used the ratio (Figure 4). The golden ratio is found in people, animals, flowers, trees, geometry, art, and architecture. It's found in the wings of a butterfly (Figure 5), the curves of a nautilus shell, the size and shape of the Parthenon. Even the double helix structure of a DNA molecule follows these proportions, perhaps explaining why we are so drawn to this ratio—it's literally in our genes.

Plastic surgeons learn about the golden ratio early in their training, as it's a very helpful way to teach them how to assess the correct relationship of length and proportion within individual facial features (such as the lips) or the relationship of different features to each other (such as the eyes to the eyebrows). In fact, a California-based maxillofacial surgeon named Stephen Marquardt derived a perfect—or rather, a perfectly *proportioned*—face from the golden ratio. He refers to it as the Golden Mask,[3] and by superimposing this mask onto an image of a face that isn't quite balanced, it allows surgeons to

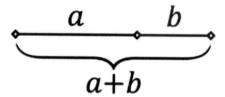

Figure 4: The golden ratio, represented by the Greek letter φ, describes a mathematical relationship between two measurements that is present in beautiful things (e.g., nature, architecture, the human body). If we think of these two measurements represented as a line AB, we can divide it at a point in the line that creates a ratio of 1.618 (A) to 1 (B), or φ.

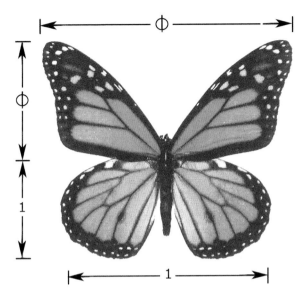

Figure 5: In nature, the golden ratio is found in the wings of a butterfly.

better pinpoint areas or features that are deficient or excessive, then illustrate their findings and their suggestions for correction or improvement to their patients (Figure 6).

Novice surgeons, as well as makeup artists, often use Golden Mean Calipers, a handy tool you can purchase online that measures the ratio of 1:1.618 on any surface (Figure 7). A great surgeon will take the golden ratio into account as one of many different factors and then use his or her aesthetic and surgical skills to make the changes the patient has requested.

Here are some guidelines for achieving a proportionate face.

EYEBROWS

The eyebrow should start in line with the inner corner of the eye. At this point, the vertical height of the eyebrow should

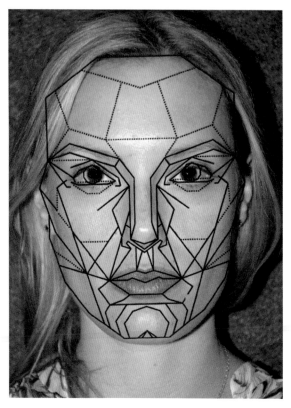

Figure 6: Marquardt's Golden Mask, which represents a perfectly proportioned face, superimposed on an attractive woman's face. Notice how her eyes, nose, cheeks, and lips have the golden ratio.

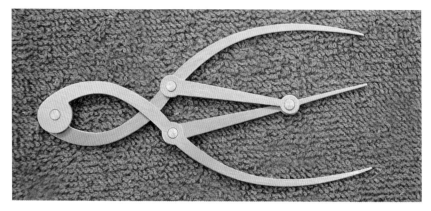

Figure 7: Golden Mean Calipers, a tool that measures the golden ratio. When the gauge is adjusted, the middle arm marks the ratio of 1:1.618 between the two lengths created.

be where the forehead bone starts. The length of the eyebrow should be 1.618 times the distance between the inner corners of the left and right eyes (this is called the intercanthal distance). There should be a gentle upward curve to the brow's lateral tip (Figure 8).

This is why many makeup artists say that eyebrows define the face—it's not so much about their thickness or shape but about their proportion. It's very easy to attain the golden ratio for your eyebrows by tweezing along their lower edge toward the lateral tip or by using an eyebrow pencil to draw in a higher brow.

This is also why people who've had a botched brow lift look so odd, as they've unwittingly been given a startled, deer-in-the-headlights look. Their eyebrows are too high in relation to

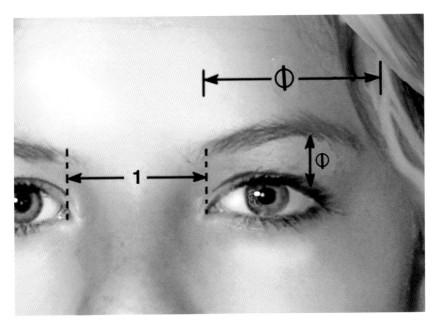

Figure 8: Beautiful eyebrow position is defined by golden proportions.

their eyes. Even if you're not trained in the golden ratio, you'll still instinctively know that something is off-kilter.

EYES AND EYELIDS

The ideal ratio for eyes is when the distance from the eyebrow at its highest outer arch to the upper eyelashes is 1.618 times the distance from the lower eyelid lashes to the beginning of the cheek. Those with rounder eyes and long lower eyelids have an inverted golden ratio, and this can be altered by high-lighting the cheeks and lower eyelids with makeup techniques (such as a smoky eye), which will shorten the appearance of the lower eyelid and create the illusion that the eye is more almond-shaped (Figure 9).

Our eyelid proportions change as we age. Older brows tend to droop over the eyes, causing the upper eyelid to shorten,

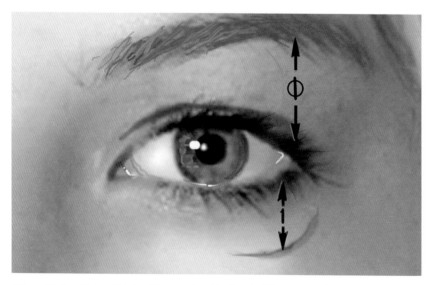

Figure 9: In beautiful, youthful eyelids, the ratio of the length of the upper to the length of the lower eyelids is φ, or 1.618.

throwing off the golden ratio. When lower eyelids and cheeks droop, the lower eyelid lengthens, reversing the beautiful proportions of the upper and lower eyelids. This change can be temporarily altered with minimally invasive techniques. Botox injections can lift the eyebrows, and fillers can shorten the length of the lower eyelid by plumping up the deep eyelid hollows and circles that make the lower eyelids appear longer. Surgery can permanently lift the brows and lower eyelids, and a mid-facelift can shorten the length of aging lower eyelids.

LIPS

One of the reasons artificially filled lips can be so jarring is because their proportions have been distorted. Overfilled lips have no *phi* relationships, and when the upper lip becomes either the same size or even larger than the lower lip, the infamous "trout pout" results. The lower lip should ideally

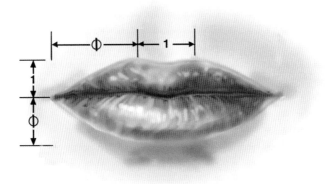

Figure 10: Beautiful lips have golden relationships within their structure.

be larger than the upper lip; in fact, according to the golden ratio, the lower lip should be 1.618 times larger than the upper lip. The distance from the two highest points of the upper lip, called peaks or a cupid's bow, to the corner of the mouth should be 1.618 times the distance between the center of the upper and lower lips (Figure 10).

This ratio is helpful when you're applying lipstick and want your lips to be naturally beautiful. And, of course, a deft hand with temporary fillers can also create an ideal proportion between top and bottom lips.

CHEEKS

Beautiful cheeks are defined by their height and volume. One of the most common requests that plastic surgeons hear is for high cheekbones—the volume of the luscious apple cheeks we had as children but with a pronounced definition. The golden ratio for cheeks can be identified by drawing a triangle from the corner of the mouth to the outer corner of the eye to the center of the ear and then drawing a line from the corner of the eye to the base of this triangle. A high cheekbone should have its apex at a ratio of 1:1.618 along this line (Figure 11).

Try doing this with some blush or bronzer, and you might be amazed at how it will make your cheekbones more defined and draw more attention to your eyes. A filler like Voluma can plump up and define cheeks, which creates the illusion that the entire face has been lifted. A stem cell facelift (fat transfers) or custom cheek implants can do this as well.

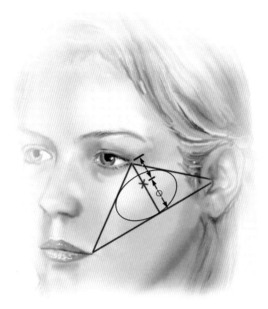

Figure 11: The apex of the ideal cheekbone should lie along a line drawn from the base of the triangle to the corner of the eye.

VOLUME

Why do youthful faces have a more appealing look than older faces? Because their golden ratio is more evident. Typically, the width between the cheekbones is approximately 1.618 times wider than the horizontal distance across the face between the right and left aspects of the chin. This creates a heart-shaped face with the most volume evident around the cheeks. As we age, however, jowls form on either side of the chin, making this horizontal length wider, and at the same time, the cheeks deflate and the distance between them decreases. You can almost think of a young cheek like a helium balloon just after it has been inflated. It is shiny, smooth, round, and full.

Eventually, the balloon slowly loses its helium and becomes nothing more than a deflated shell. As this deflation of the cheeks occurs, the aging face becomes more square shaped and less heart shaped. My female patients often tell me that when this happens, they suddenly look more masculine. Injectable hyaluronic acid fillers can be added to the upper cheeks as a quick treatment to restore more of a heart-shaped proportion, especially for patients in their forties.

As we age further, the cheeks lose more volume, the jowls become bigger and heavier, and the face becomes shaped like an inverted heart, almost like a triangle. For older patients, using fillers to replace this lost volume doesn't work as well as it does for those in their thirties and forties. Adding extra filler to the cheeks converts this inverted triangle into a facial square, stacking volume in the middle and upper face over an already widened lower face with jowls. This creates the wide and stuffed appearance we associate with an overfilled face. Furthermore, because our faces become looser and less sup-portive as we age, the added weight of these fillers will make the cheeks droop further, creating an almost simian or ape-like appearance. Actress Courteney Cox admitted to using facial fillers in the cheeks around the time she turned fifty years old but then reversed them (getting them dissolved away) because they created an unnaturally wide and altering look to her face.[4] This is why people who continue getting filler when they're in their fifties and sixties often look fake or plastic. For older patients who want to restore volume and rejuvenate their faces, a facelift is the best solution and will lift the widened

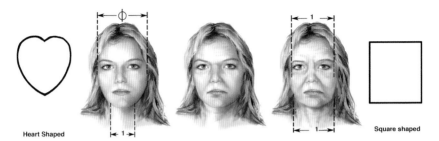

Figure 12: Youth is represented by a heart-shaped face with the width along the apex of the cheekbones 1.618 the distance between the right and left aspects of the chin. Aging results in deflation of the cheek region and widening of the area around the chin, with the formation of jowls creating a more square-shaped face where the ratio between the upper and lower face is 1:1.

and heavy jowls back up over the cheeks turning the inverted triangle back to the heart-shaped face of youth (Figure 12).

I hope these guidelines will help you better understand the science behind beauty and aging and how proportion can impact your face. In the next part, I'll tell you how to harness this information to find the best surgeon for the procedures and techniques that will produce the results you are looking for. The more information you have, the more likely you will achieve a positive, successful plastic surgery experience.

1 Doug Jones and Kim Hill, "Criteria of Facial Attractiveness in Five Populations," *Human Nature* 4, no. 3 (1993), 271–296, doi: 10.1007/BF02692202, https://www.ncbi.nlm.nih.gov/pubmed/24214367.

2 Judith H. Langlois et al., "Infant Preferences for Attractive Faces: Rudiments of a Stereotype?" *Developmental Psychology* 23, no. 3 (1987), 363–369, http://psycnet.apa.org/record/1987-24635-001.

3 Eugene L. Gottlieb and Stephen R. Marquardt, "JCO Interviews Dr. Stephen R. Marquardt on the Golden Decagon and Human Facial Beauty," *Journal of Clinical Orthodontics*, June 2002, https://www.jco-online.com/archive/2002/06/339-jco-interviews-dr-stephen-r-marquardt-on-the-golden-decagon-and-human-facial-beauty/.

4 Cortney Pellettieri, "Courteney Cox Gets Candid," *New Beauty*, June 22, 2017, https://www.newbeauty.com/blog/dailybeauty/11013-courteney-cox-beauty/.

PART
II

PLASTIC SURGERY 101:
THE BASICS

3

Quacks, Scams, and Botched Faces

How to Avoid Becoming a Plastic Surgery Victim

It's strange when patients come to my office seeking help that they're actually terrified to accept. People visiting cosmetic surgeons for the first time have a lot of fears. They fear the risk of anesthesia. They fear infection. They fear complications during surgery. They fear pain and long recoveries. They fear scarring and deformity. They fear that they will look like one of those horror slideshows of celebrity plastic surgery gone terribly wrong.

They fear less dramatic consequences, too. They fear that they won't look like themselves anymore. They fear they will not like the results. They fear wasting thousands of dollars on something that won't work. They fear the dreaded "plastic surgery addiction"—if they do it once, will they be unable to stop?

And they fear that people will know they did it. A recent *New York Times* editorial by journalist Joyce Wadler described this fear and the lengths to which she went to make sure nobody knew she was recovering from a facelift.[1] As she points out, people talk openly about other surgeries and procedures. They talk about their personal lives, their beauty regimes, even their sex lives. They admit when they have surgery after an accident or to cure a medical problem, but nobody talks about their plastic surgery.

All these fears are perfectly understandable, and many of them are completely legitimate. You might experience negative effects in your life if plastic surgery results are obvious or if they change your look too substantially. A recent survey from England revealed that 20 percent of respondents who had plastic surgery were unhappy with the results and 50 percent said they felt pressured into doing procedures by their doctor or their doctor's staff.[2] Some surgeons aren't very good at making their results look natural or guiding their patients toward the results that are most likely to work best on their faces and for their issues. Some procedures don't do much, if anything, and cost a lot of money. Some people are shocked by the recovery time, or the way they look right after surgery, simply because they didn't know what was coming. There are also some studies that show that people who suffer from depression, anxiety, or body dysmorphia disorder are more likely to be dissatisfied with any plastic surgery results.[3]

I have to admit that doing revisions of botched or otherwise problematic work, while extremely rewarding, is difficult. The initial surgery always leaves scar tissue, complicating my ability to mold and restore the tissues. Revision patients often have a protracted recuperation with longer healing times. This is why it is so important for you to do any and every procedure properly the first time. It's always worth the additional effort to find the right doctor, and it could be worth the additional money that the best doctor might charge. If you try to cut corners, you may eventually spend three times as much on repairs and corrections as you would have for one well-researched procedure done right the first time—revisions are always more expensive. I feel terrible for the revision plastic surgery patients I see in consultation who could have saved themselves pain, suffering, huge fees, wasted time, and the emotional trauma of having to live with a botched procedure for up to a year. Yes, one whole year! For most plastic surgery revisions, the face needs to heal for a minimum of a year in order for the blood supply to completely return to the operated area to allow for proper healing.

But here's the thing—when performed by an experienced and ethical physician, facial enhancement procedures are very safe. Most people who get plastic surgery are happy with the results and say it was worth the money and time. And if you know how to choose the right surgeon and research your procedure, then you won't be surprised by anything. You will be going into your procedure—whether it is something very minor like Botox or something pretty major like a facelift—armed with full knowledge and realistic expectations.

This chapter will show you exactly what to avoid so that you never have to be afraid, so that you never end up with a doctor you don't trust or a procedure that you didn't even want. Most importantly, this chapter will outline everything you need to know to make sure your results are natural. If you follow these steps, the only way anyone will ever know you've had plastic surgery is if you decide to tell them.

Step One: Take Your Internal Temperature

Before you make an appointment for a consultation with a physician, you should ask yourself: Am I a good candidate for plastic surgery? The way to answer this question is by taking your internal temperature. It's part of your due diligence. You can do all the research you want and follow the steps I'm about to lay out to a T—but none of that matters if your internal temperature is too hot.

If you are experiencing a great deal of psychological or emotional unrest in your life, it is not a good time to pursue plastic surgery. I see this over and over again—patients come in and tell me they've just lost their job, or found out their spouse is cheating, or they were recently divorced, or there's been a death in the family. Choosing to have plastic surgery during these situations is a very reactive decision. Often, patients are looking for something that will give them immediate gratification or take the pain away. They assume that changing their appearance will change their whole lives. Unfortunately, after surgery they remain the same people, with the same needs— just with new noses or crisper jawlines.

Other times patients come to see me and admit that they are being pressured to have plastic surgery by other people, which is a huge red flag. I ask them how they genuinely feel about their appearance and try to dissuade them from surgery. You should always be true to yourself.

Another red flag is whenever a new patient rushes in and wants to get a procedure done immediately. It is always best to take time making this decision, as with all other important decisions in our lives, so that it is not reactive or hasty. Most often, the patients who feel that their procedures have been successful are the same patients who deliberated, taking time before they decided to pursue surgery. These patients do their research. They make lists. They weigh the pros and cons.

Before you do anything else, let your internal temperature cool down to normal. Ask yourself: What is my motivation for this surgery, really? Am I having any doubts? Am I feeling pressured? Do I want to have this procedure because it will show my cheating ex what they're missing? Do I feel that not having this procedure is holding me back from the next thing that I'm looking for in my life? Do I believe that my whole life will be better after this surgery? If the answer to any of the questions on this list except the first is yes, then take a step back. Wait a while.

Plastic surgery is not a magical gateway to a perfect life. Even if your surgery makes you more youthful or attractive, if you don't take care of your mental health and emotional needs, the external conditions in your life are not going to change. I've had patients come in and tell me they spent $8,000 on fillers for their face from another doctor, and that while they are satisfied with the physical results, they're still disappointed, even miserable, to find that none of the big life changes they expected have occurred. On the other hand, I have also treated patients with just one Botox shot who are thrilled to pieces afterward to see that the line between their eyes that had made them look angry all the time has finally disappeared. The intended outcomes in these two situations are quite different.

Before you book a consultation, take your internal temperature again. Ask yourself: Do I want to have this procedure so I can have more confidence about some aspect of my appearance that has been bothering me for a long time? Do I want to look my best for an important upcoming life event? If both answers are yes, great. These are excellent reasons to have plastic surgery.

One of my favorite patients to treat was a woman who was getting ready for her child's wedding. She was in a good place, looking forward to sharing in her family's happiness. She just wanted a little bit of an edge for the blessed event. She came in and told me what she wanted and why. She had the support of her partner and the rest of her family. She was not anxious, just exhilarated. She had realistic expectations, she was relaxed, and she was in the best possible emotional place. She got it done, she healed well, and she moved on.

Step Two: Don't Be the First One on the Bandwagon

Never, ever try any new technique, device, or procedure that has only been available or on the market for less than one year. I can't tell you how many brand-new, supposedly game-changing techniques and products have come onto the market only to completely disappear a year later when real-world application has proved to be disastrous.

Over the last ten years, hundreds of products have come and gone. This happens in particular with a lot of injectables, lasers, and other devices. First, they get cleared by the FDA, which endorses safety but not efficacy—in other words, the FDA doesn't say that the product or device actually does anything, only that it probably won't hurt you. Then, the manufacturer has to do a whole lot of marketing and publicity to get people to use the product to recoup the hundreds of millions of dollars they spent going through that legally necessary FDA approval process. If they want to make their money back, they'd better make that product sound practically miraculous.

A good example of this phenomenon is a device called Thermage. This facial-tightening treatment was presented on the *Oprah Winfrey Show* in 2003, spurring cosmetic surgeons all over the country to buy Thermage machines throughout the 2000s. But the product did nothing to tighten faces or necks, as its advertisements and representatives had promised. I remember the fallout clearly, because many of the people who'd spent thousands of dollars on this treatment came into my office seeking plastic surgery after realizing that Thermage was a dud.

During that crucial first year on the market, as more and more people experience a new product or device and go online to rate it or post comments about it, you'll be able to find either a lot of praise about how well it works or a lot of backlash about how poorly it works. After a year, many products and devices will no longer be available because they've gone out of business. Or maybe the new product, device, technique, or procedure is a game changer and after the first year is still going strong. But either way, you won't know much for about a year, and that year's worth of public feedback is extremely valuable information for you. Before you try something new, you want to know how others have fared. Twelve months of feedback will tell you that.

I'm not saying you shouldn't engage with new technology, which can be exciting and groundbreaking. All I'm saying is don't engage with brand-new technology. Don't jump on the bandwagon prematurely. Give it a year, monitor the progress, and, if all signs point to success, you can feel much more comfortable about giving it a try.

Step Three: If It's on TV at Midnight (or Any Time), Step Away from Your Credit Card

One of the easiest and best ways to avoid getting scammed is to never, ever buy a product or device advertised on TV that promises to reverse facial aging. None of them work. I'm sorry to burst any bubbles, but no matter how amazing it looks, or how fantastic the results appear on the models, there simply is not, nor will there ever be, an effective anti-aging device that is sold legally "over the counter." TV marketers can be geniuses in generating excitement about a product, but it is all false advertising. Commercials can lie, and they *do* lie.

A classic example is a spring device heavily advertised throughout the 1990s that you were supposed to hold between your chin and neck and flex, almost like a bicep curl. The theory was that this would tighten the neck because it strengthened the neck muscles. The commercial showed how easy it was, and the beautiful models showed off their firm necks and curvaceous chins. However, I am here to tell you that those models' firm necks had absolutely nothing to do with the hokey and completely ineffectual device.

Facial tissue sags not because your neck muscles are weak but because they have been stretched out by gravity and age. No matter how much you exercise them, they are not going to get any tighter. In fact, if you over-flex your facial muscles too often, you'll actually only succeed in further loosening the skin and creating more wrinkles, so devices like this can actually have the *opposite* effect of the advertised result.

If a device has actually been proven to reverse signs of facial aging, it should be available in your physician's office. If it is sold over the counter, without a prescription, there is absolutely no burden of legal proof that it has to work. Just as with the FDA, which makes sure things are sufficiently safe but does not do anything to guarantee efficacy, it is not required that any noninvasive, nonsurgical anti-aging device go through any legal or scientific process to prove it works.

What's more, the only products or procedures that manipulate tissues in a deeper fashion, that actually make a visible change in sagging and wrinkles, are all regulated and require a medical professional to administer. It's easy to understand why everybody is looking for a less expensive, less invasive way to look younger. But when it comes to facial aging, the simple fact is that the anatomical changes that occur at the level of the skin, including thinning and stretching, simply cannot be reversed by any kind of external treatment that would be safe to sell without a doctor's involvement.

Step Four: Ask Others for Good Recommendations

Use your smarts and connections. If you have friends or family members who have had surgery themselves, or who know others who have, they can give you some direction. Ask your family doctor who is reputable in your community. If they don't know anyone, they can call a colleague who does. Try to get a referral from somebody in the field. I get this request often from prospective patients, especially from those who live out of town or who know I only do plastic surgery on the face. They'll tell me that they can't make the trip to New York but ask me whom I would trust to do this procedure in Chicago or Florida or Texas. Or they ask me whom might I recommend in New York for a breast augmentation or a tummy tuck. You can always call or email a plastic surgeon's office with your questions.

Step Five: Use RealSelf.com as a Resource

These days, there are review sites for everybody and everything. Yelp was one of the first, when it began offering a platform publishing user-generated restaurant reviews. Now, just about every product and service available in the world has reviews online, but the most useful, free resource for anyone considering cosmetic surgery is a website called RealSelf.com.

RealSelf is a community for consumers of plastic surgery treatments of all types and levels, and the number of people on this site is quite large. Users rate and describe treatments, products, and physicians. From acne scar removal to skin lightening, chemical peels to lip augmentation, fat transfers to hair transplants, you can get detailed firsthand information about what the experience was like for other patients, often with graphic photos. If you are considering any type of plastic surgery, the wealth of information on this behemoth of a website is invaluable. Whether it is Botox, CoolSculpting, or Ultherapy, you won't just hear about whether or not something works. You will also get detailed descriptions of others' entire experiences—what they did, how much it hurt, how it looked right afterward, how it looked after healing, and whether they think they got their money's worth. RealSelf is also a very helpful platform for consumers who have questions. As soon as a question is posted, dozens of surgeons from all over the United States individually respond; it's almost like getting a free consultation from home.

Members say the site is addictive—once you go down the rabbit hole, you can waste hours of time reading stories and looking at photos. But if you are legitimately considering a procedure or product, I highly recommend going down the rabbit hole; unlike most internet deep-dives, this will be time well spent. The more you read, the more you will understand about your procedure. Plus, you'll be able to view real (and sometimes raw) photographic evidence of the experience. This can help you decide if you really want to do what you were planning. Maybe you will realize that it will be totally worthwhile. Or maybe you will realize that you aren't willing to go through what others describe or that what you've heard about a product is more hype than reality. The important thing is that you've gathered a lot of information you didn't have before.

Step Six: Read Reviews

After you've perused RealSelf.com and have narrowed your search to one or more doctors, look up their practices on physician review sites such as RateMDs, Healthgrades, and Vitals for feedback from current or former patients.

All reviews posted directly on a physician's website are handpicked and, of course, positive. Impartial review sites will give you a more honest accounting. Be critical of everything you read on these sites but realize that if most posts describe a similar experience, they're more than likely truthful. Consider the number of reviews, too: Hundreds of reviews probably reflect a lot more experience than just a couple of reviews, which may reveal a surgeon newly in practice. Are the reviews overwhelmingly positive? Mixed? Overwhelmingly negative? A few outlying bad reviews amongst many positive ones are normal, but multiple bad reviews are definitely a red flag. Remember that reviews will describe not only the outcomes of specific procedures but also the quality of the staff and the personality of the doctor, which can greatly impact your experience.

Look carefully at which procedures are reviewed. If, for example, you're seeking a rhinoplasty but you see that 90 percent of a surgeon's reviews discuss his or her skill at breast augmentation and only a handful mention other procedures, you can deduce that noses aren't this surgeon's specialty. In that case, perhaps you should consider a different surgeon.

Step Seven: Choose a Specialist and Fully Vet Your Surgeon

In the world of cosmetic surgery, core specialties are extremely important. You wouldn't go to your family practice doctor for brain surgery—you'd go to a brain surgeon. If you need a facial procedure, you should go to a specialist in facial procedures (whether surgical or nonsurgical), or, even better, a specialist in the kind of specific facial surgery you need, such as a rhinoplasty or eye surgery.

But it isn't enough just to look for a physician or surgeon who is "board certified," because different organizations have different levels of requirements for earning that designation. For some, you need only take a couple of courses and an exam before being allowed to advertise yourself as a "board-certified surgeon," without ever having to complete a surgical residency.

Any doctor could get this certification without putting in the clinical hours that represent real surgical specialty experience.

Other organizations, however, require much more training and experience. Currently, there are five different legitimate boards that are either members of the American Board of Medical Specialties (ABMS) or found equivalent to the ABMS: the American Board of Facial Plastic and Reconstructive Surgery; the American Board of Plastic Surgery; the American Board of Dermatology; the American Board of Otolaryngology/Head and Neck Surgery; and the American Board of Ophthalmology.

I am a board-certified and fellowship-trained facial plastic surgeon, which means that I completed five years of an Otolaryngology/Head and Neck Surgery residency, during which I only operated on the face, nose, eyelids, head, and neck. During this time, I performed cancer surgeries for the head, neck, nose, and face, including reconstructive surgery on the face, as well as cosmetic procedures such as rhinoplasty, eyelid lifts, and facelifts. I then went on to complete an additional year of fellowship training through the American Academy of Facial Plastic and Reconstructive Surgery, specializing further in the most updated techniques in facial plastic and reconstructive surgery. Any surgeon who lists these credentials has completed the same level of training.

However, board certification, though important, is just the beginning. Cosmetic surgery is both a skill and an art; just because a doctor has all the required credentials doesn't necessarily mean that he or she will be able to create the look you desire.

Every type of plastic surgery requires a high level of expertise. The plastic surgeon you are considering should have already performed hundreds or even thousands of procedures like the one you want. He or she should have at least five years (preferably ten) of experience in that area and should be able to show you many before-and-after examples of good and consistent results. These results should present patients whose facial architecture and skin type are the same as yours. The more surgeons do the same procedure, the more they will fine-tune and improve their techniques. Surgeons who only occasionally perform a procedure will not have the same level of skill as those who do it all the time.

CHECK HOSPITAL AFFILIATIONS

The next item on your checklist should be your doctor's hospital affiliations. If a physician has privileges to perform surgery at an accredited hospital, this demonstrates that his or her performance and credentials are subject to regular scrutiny. While most plastic surgeons perform surgery only in their offices, they should also have privileges to perform surgery at a local hospital, in case a long and complicated surgery is needed. If a doctor does not have these privileges, seek someone else who does.

CONFIRM THAT YOUR SURGEON'S IN-OFFICE OPERATING SUITE IS ACCREDITED

The operating room in which your plastic surgery is planned should be an accredited facility overseen by one of three

different organizations: American Association for Accreditation of Ambulatory Surgery Facilities (AAAASF), Joint
Commission on Accreditation of Healthcare Organizations
(JCAHO), or Accreditation Association for Ambulatory
Health Care (AAAHC). Accreditation ensures that equipment
is up to date, emergency supplies and medications are available, and staff is adequately trained and licensed.

I believe it is preferable to have your surgery performed
in your surgeon's office. Why? Hospitals are colonized with
antibiotic-resistant bacteria, including the staph infection
MRSA, which theoretically increases the risk of contamina-
tion for surgical patients who are exposed to them. Another
benefit of in-office surgery is privacy. In a hospital, you are
one patient among dozens having surgery that day, but in your
plastic surgeon's office, the care and attention is focused on
you.

ASK ABOUT ANESTHESIA

If you are having anesthesia, ask about the credentials of your
future anesthesiologist. I only use physicians who are board-
certified anesthesiologists. Many patients have questions about
the type of anesthesia that will be performed and the related
risks, and I put them in touch directly with my anesthesiologist,
whose answers will be expert and specific. I discuss the options
for anesthesia in more detail in Chapter 12.

Never, Ever Have Any Procedures Done Outside of an Accredited Medical Facility

Priscilla Presley is an incredibly beautiful and wealthy woman. Yet even she, a smart and savvy businesswoman, ended up with a botched face when an Argentinian doctor (without a license to practice in the United States) came to her privately and injected her with low-grade industrial silicone—the kind used to lubricate cars.[4]

Why did she choose to do this when she could have gone to any of the best plastic surgeons or cosmetic dermatologists in the world? I can't answer that. But I do know that there are a lot of people who fall prey to quacks who charge enormous sums of money to make house calls.

Bottom line: If you want a medical procedure of any kind, have it done in a sterile environment by a thoroughly vetted professional. Do not go to a Botox party at your friend's house, no matter how trendy and fun the Botox-wielder allegedly is. Do not cut financial corners with someone who gives you a "discount" if they come to you. You are setting yourself up for a problem, even a disaster. Chances are, you'll have to pay later for someone else to undo the damage done.

Step Eight: Look at Online Before-and-After Photographs with a Critical Eye

In this age of digital communication, experienced and reputable physicians should have detailed information on their websites, including before-and-after photos. If you are considering rhinoplasty from a specific doctor, look at the pictures of the noses the surgeon has done. How often does your doctor perform the surgery that you need, and are the outcomes positive? Does his or her site include many rhinoplasty pictures, or only one or two, compared to other procedures?

Before-and-after photos also provide a huge clue about the surgeon's personal aesthetic. Does it match yours? If every rhinoplasty picture on the doctor's site reveals a sloping, piggy, or pinched nose, then you can assume that you will probably get something similar. If that's not what you want, don't go with that surgeon, even if he or she has all the right degrees and certifications.

Not all physicians are in tune to their patients' desires. Some even practice assembly-line surgeries, giving each of their patients the same nose or eyes or cheeks or neck, regardless of request or description. Imagine a stylist is going to choose a dress for you. Maybe he or she really likes green sleeveless dresses, but you hate green and you like sleeves. If that's the case, then no matter how beautiful that green sleeveless dress might look to your stylist, or to everyone else, you aren't going to be happy with it because it doesn't match your personal style.

There are two things to look for in before-and-afters. First, the "before" photo should be taken with the same lighting, the same makeup, and with the face in the same exact position as the "after" photo. That is the only way you can make a valid comparison between the two. Second, it's very important to find a physician who can modify their aesthetic. The patients in the before-and-after photos should not all look the same, but they should all look balanced. Results depend on gender, ethnicity, and personal choice. Varied results are evidence of a good surgeon who can fine-tune and modify outcomes rather than produce assembly-line features.

Your physician should also allow you to speak or meet with other patients who have had the surgery you are interested in. We do this all the time at my office, and it's even better than a photograph for the new patient because they can see a living, breathing example of our results. You can get a live account of that person's experience with the surgery, the outcome, the recovery, the staff, and the demeanor of the physician, and you can ask questions. I would be wary of any office that refuses to let you speak to former patients.

Step Nine: Be Vigilant During Your Consultation

Your next step is to schedule a consultation. It's a good idea to come in with a written list of questions so you don't forget anything. There's a lot to talk about, and I'm always glad to see that a prospective patient has already done his or her homework before we start talking. I encourage my prospective patients to have multiple consultations with different surgeons. This will not only give you answers to your medical questions, but it will help you make an informed decision about whom you like best. See as many doctors as you need to see. Some of my patients have seen six or seven surgeons, multiple times, over many years, before they finally make their decision. There's no magic formula.

PAY ATTENTION TO THE OFFICE ENVIRONMENT

If you choose to have surgery with this doctor, you will be spending quite a bit of time in the office, so it is crucial that you feel comfortable there.

Do you feel welcome? Is the front-desk staff courteous and professional? Is the waiting room comfortable? Is the bathroom spotless? Are you offered a cold drink or a hot coffee? Even if you're happy and excited to be discussing a procedure you've wanted for a long time, sitting in a doctor's office is always going to produce some level of stress, so your visit should be as pleasant as possible.

EXPECT COURTEOUS AND DETAILED ANSWERS TO ALL YOUR QUESTIONS

The consultation is for your benefit. A good doctor will listen to your concerns, answer all your questions, and explain all the risks and benefits of the procedures you are interested in. If the surgeon does not give you adequate time or becomes frustrated when you ask detailed questions, it's safe to assume that he or she will probably not be supportive after surgery.

USE PHOTOGRAPHS TO DESCRIBE WHAT YOU WANT

You need to be as detailed as possible when describing what you want. They say a picture is worth a thousand words, and this is especially true with plastic surgery! I suggest using Google Images to find faces that resemble yours but that feature the characteristic that you'd like to have. This will make your preferences clear, from your general aesthetic to your specific desired result. If you are coming in to discuss a rejuvenating procedure, bring photos of your younger self so that the surgeon understands how aging has affected your face. Images of your more youthful face will help the surgeon decide what procedures will be best for you.

TAKE ADVANTAGE OF DIGITAL MORPHING

It is helpful for surgeons to use digital morphing programs to simulate the changes you can expect with your procedure. This allows you and the surgeon to confer on what you want, and you can work together as a team to create your desired outcome. If the surgeon's aesthetic does not match yours, it will be evident in the morphing.

DON'T FALL FOR THE BAIT AND SWITCH

This happens when you come in for one procedure and the surgeon tries to sell you something else entirely that conforms to his or her preferences and not yours. If you ask for a rhinoplasty and the surgeon tries to convince you to augment your cheeks, get out of there. Focus on what you're worried about. There are certain cases when one procedure might be enhanced by another; for example, if you have a large nose and a small chin, reducing your nose and augmenting your chin might bring about more facial harmony—but that does not mean you have to do both procedures. Improving one part of your face doesn't mean you have to improve all parts of your face. Remember that you can always come back and do something else later.

I once had a consultation with a forty-year-old woman who had gone to someone else for her nose but had wound up getting a brow lift, a chin implant, and fat grafting. "It's been six months, and I don't look like myself," she said to me in tears. She didn't look bad; her surgeon did a good job, but it just wasn't what she was originally looking for. Don't let this happen to you!

After your consultation is over, and if you decide to go ahead with your procedure, you will meet with a patient care coordinator. The coordinator will discuss financing, book your surgery dates, give you detailed pre- and post-operative instructions, and answer any other questions you may have. If you're a smoker, now is the time to start cutting back (and hopefully quit entirely), as smoking has negative effects on the healing process.

Step Ten: Trust Your Gut

Last but definitely not least: Listen to your intuition. Trust your gut.

Imagine you're having a consultation with a surgeon, and you really like their office, their staff, and their personality. You've done lots of research and seen photos, and you can tell they're skillful and kind. You really want to use them because you like them, but something's off. You don't know why, but you just have one of those bad feelings. Trust that feeling and move on. If anything feels off to you, don't do it! You can always make another appointment in a few months and see if you get the same gut feeling.

Often, patients make a destination trip to the surgeon they think will be "the one." They take the day off work to come to New York City and meet a doctor who's got a big reputation. And because of the effort they've already expended, the time they've already spent, they then force themselves into going through with a preconceived plan, despite not feeling 100 percent sure they're making the right decision. My suggestion is to put all of your expectations aside when you walk into the office and instead try to concentrate on being open-minded. Ask your questions and listen carefully to the answers. Take notes. Look at lots of before-and-after photos.

And then, even if everything else seems right, if at the very last moment before you make your final decision you have any hesitation—not about the procedure, not about being scared about surgery, but a feeling in your gut that tells you that there's something off about the person you're about to entrust with your face, your body, your life—stop right there and say no. Don't give the surgeon a pass just because he has received impressive accolades or has a big practice or famous clients. There should never be any hesitation.

Why is this so important? Because you need to have an emotional connection not only with your surgeon but also with the staff, with the space, and with the whole experience. It's a wholly intangible part of the process, but personality is important. Some surgeons are brilliant technicians but very clinical and sterile, and you might find that off-putting (while someone with the same kind of gruffness might find it appealingly comfortable and familiar). This is why, if you were given the choice between three top surgeons, all of whom get good results and have stellar reputations, the best decision will be for you to go with the surgeon you personally like the best— the surgeon who makes you feel comfortable and puts you at ease. You don't want to have to go through the process all over again when you're forced to see someone new for a revision. Listen to your gut. When you do, you'll make the right choice.

This is just the beginning. This is my primary, first line of advice for avoiding scams, quacks, and botched results, and for saving your hard-earned money to spend on what actually works. In each subsequent chapter in this book, you'll learn more about what to watch out for, what doesn't work, and what will waste your money and time.

Are you ready to get serious? Are you ready for transformation? Let's begin with your skin.

1 Joyce Wadler, "Swear You Will Tell No One," *New York Times*, May 4, 2017, https://www. nytimes.com/2017/05/04/nyregion/hiding-cosmetic-surgery-bias.html.

2 Lauren Paxman, "Costly Mistake: One in Five Who Have Plastic Surgery Are Unhappy with the Results," Treatment Advisor via *Daily Mail*, October 19, 2011, http://www.dailymail.co.uk/femail/ article-2050938/Costly-mistake-One-plastic-surgery-unhappy-results.html.

3 Megan M. Kelly, Elizabeth R. Didie, and Ashley S. Hart, "Cosmetic Treatments and Body Dysmorphic Disorder," International OCD Foundation, https://bdd.iocdf.org/expert-opinions/ cosmetic-treatments-and-bdd.

4 Robert Kotler, "Priscilla Presley and Silicone," *WebMD Second Opinion: Secrets of a Beverly Hills Cosmetic Surgeon*, April 11, 2008, https://blogs.webmd.com/cosmetic-surgery/2008/04/priscilla-presley-and-silicone.html.

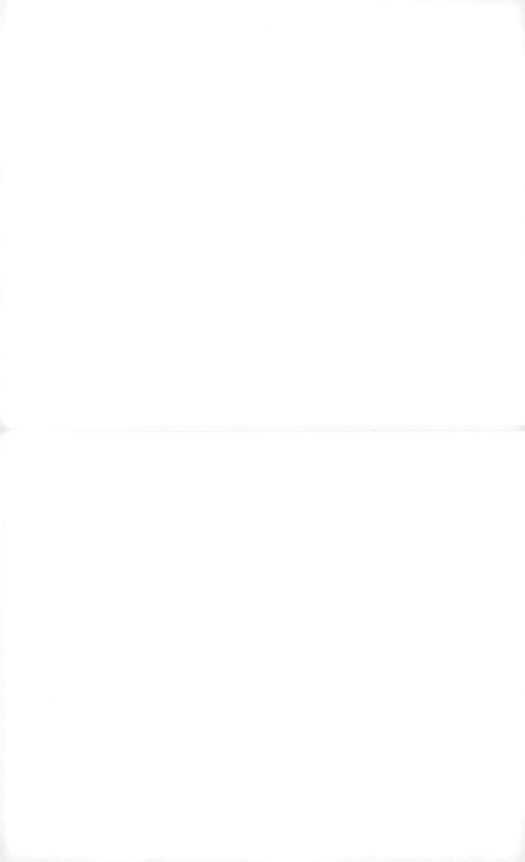

4

Begin with the Skin

No matter what plastic surgery procedure you might be considering, or what skin-care concerns you have, before you book your first appointment with any practitioner, it's very important to understand the fundamental facts about your skin and how it changes as you get older. The more you know, the less money, time, and energy you'll waste on overhyped products and treatments.

We are all seeking the fountain of youth in a jar. Consumers are willing to spend hundreds, even thousands, of dollars a year on creams, masks, and serums in attempts to stave off the inevitable. Anyone who has ever walked into Sephora or into the cosmetic section of a department store knows just how true this is. Unfortunately, many highly touted ingredients in over-the-counter skin-care products have never been shown to work from a clinical trial perspective.

My goal in this section is to educate you on the ingredients in skin-care products that really do work. It's not a long list, but if you understand active ingredients and their effects, you can avoid expensive fads and products that sound too good to be true (as they almost always are) and spend your hard-earned money only on the ones that are genuinely worth it. Eventually, however, even the most effective topical products cease to make a major difference in wrinkles, hyperpigmentation, and thinning of the skin. When this happens, it may be time to seek out physician-administered resurfacing treatments like peels and lasers. This chapter will also define and describe these procedures so that you can choose what is most appropriate for your skin type, age, and condition.

Skin Fundamentals

Your skin is the largest organ of your body and consists of three layers: the epidermis, the dermis, and the deeper subcutaneous tissue (Figure 13). The epidermis is the topmost skin layer. It is covered by a protective layer of dead skin cells called the stratum corneum, which acts like armor to retain your skin's moisture and oils. The stratum corneum is shed continuously and replaced with new cells from the deepest layer of the epidermis, called the basal cell layer. As we age, it takes longer for the stratum corneum to shed and renew itself. The epidermis becomes thicker, causing the skin to feel and look rough and dry. Sun exposure and smoking also accelerate the aging process.

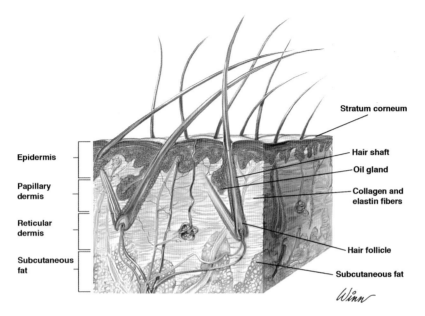

Epidermis

Papillary
dermis

Reticular
dermis

Subcutaneous
fat

Stratum corneum

Hair shaft

Oil gland

Collagen and
elastin fibers

Hair follicle

Subcutaneous fat

Winn

Figure 13: The three layers of the skin: epidermis, dermis, and subcutaneous fat layer.

The dermis makes up about 80 percent of the thickness of the skin and is its workhorse. It contains sebaceous glands, hair follicles, sweat glands, blood vessels, and nerve sensors that allow us to feel light touch, temperature, and pain. All of these structures are enmeshed in a dense network of collagen and elastin (elastic fibers), the primary proteins that support the skin and give it strength and elasticity. As we age, this collagen layer decreases and the elastin fibers become fragmented and disorganized, accounting for the thinner appearance of the skin in older faces.

Under the epidermis and dermis is a layer composed mostly of fibrous tissue and fat called the subcutaneous tissue. Its function is to insulate the body and further protect the organs— think of it as a shock absorber of sorts. This helps keep the skin plump and smooth. The loss of fat that naturally occurs with age results in depressions in the skin causing the skin to sag and fold; additional damage occurs with sun exposure and smoking.

INTRINSIC AND EXTRINSIC AGING

There are many visible signs of aging skin: an uneven complexion, loss of radiance, dry and rough patches, enlarged pores, pigmentation spots, lines and wrinkles, sagging, sallowness, broken capillaries, and skin growths.

Skin ages in two ways: intrinsic and extrinsic. Intrinsic aging is what you can't control: your genes, your ethnicity, and any inherent diseases or medical conditions. Extrinsic aging, on the other hand, is what you *can* control with your lifestyle. This includes how much time you spend in the sun, whether or not you smoke or drink, how healthy your diet is, and other daily habits. You can prevent extrinsic aging by avoiding skin pollutants/wrinkle generators, protecting your skin from daily sun exposure, and supplementing and nourishing your skin with prescriptive skin care that actually works to help maintain your skin's suppleness.

WRINKLE GENERATORS

There are four major wrinkle generators: sun exposure, smoking, excessive alcohol intake, and poor nutrition.

1. **Sun exposure:** There is no such thing as a healthy tan and there never will be. The rate of skin cancer is higher

than ever primarily because people ignore the need for daily skin protection from the sun. If sun exposure doesn't give you cancer, unhealthy tanning will certainly give you wrinkles. Worse, sun exposure causes the production of unstable and harmful molecules called free radicals that can damage virtually every part of a cell, including its DNA. In fact, these scavenging particles are believed to be the major culprit with respect to aging, heart disease, and cancer. Free radicals are produced as a normal function of the energy process, but sun exposure accelerates and accentuates them.

2. **Smoking:** There is nothing good to say about smoking. You already know how bad it is for your overall health and well-being, to say nothing of what secondhand smoke does to everyone in a smoker's orbit. What you may not know is that smoking has especially harmful effects on the skin. Nicotine causes blood vessels in the skin to constrict, reducing blood supply to the skin, which deprives it of nourishment. Over time, this thins all three skin layers and also causes the release of additional free radicals.

3. **Excessive alcohol intake:** Drinking too much depletes many essential nutrients, vitamins, and minerals from our bodies, including the B-vitamin complex and folate, which are essential to skin-cell reproduction and health. It also causes free radical production to increase in the bloodstream. So, while the health benefits of a

single glass of red wine at dinner have been extensively studied, drinking more than that, especially on a regular basis, will negatively affect your skin.

4. **Poor nutrition:** A diet of processed junk food depletes essential nutrients and so does an excessively restrictive diet. You need a certain amount of fat in your body for your skin to look healthy, which is why excessive dieters often look pinched and haggard, especially in their faces. Yo-yo dieting, which repeatedly expands and deflates the skin, causes sagging and additional wrinkles.

Protecting Your Skin from the Sun

In addition to avoiding wrinkle generators, we all need to protect our skin from the sun to prevent photo-aging. *Photo-aging* is the term for the long-term thinning, sagging, and wrinkling that is caused by the sun's rays. You can easily see the difference between photo-aged skin and normally aged skin if you compare the skin on your face and hands (which are exposed to sunlight every day you're outside, even if for only a few minutes) with the skin on your buttocks (which never gets exposed to the sun, unless you're wearing a tiny bikini). The difference is quite evident, isn't it?

Sunlight contains two kinds of ultraviolet (UV) light: longer, UVA rays and shorter, UVB rays. UVB rays are the main cause of sunburn and most skin cancers. UVA rays, while not as powerful, penetrate more deeply into the skin and are the chief cause of skin wrinkling, leathering, and actual damage to the DNA in your cells.

SUNSCREEN

The American Academy of Dermatology recommends that you apply a sunscreen or sunblock with a sun protection factor (SPF) of 30 or higher thirty minutes before you go outside each day. Get in the habit of applying sunscreen each morning— apply it under your moisturizer, for example, or right after you brush your teeth.

SPF measures protection against sunburn-creating UVB rays but not damaging UVA rays. If it normally takes five minutes for a sunburn to develop on a summer day, a sunscreen with an SPF rating of 30 would allow you to stay outside safely thirty times longer (150 minutes). Sunblocks that contain zinc oxide and titanium oxide also block UVA rays, which cause facial wrinkling. Always use a broad-spectrum sunscreen that contains protection against both UVA and UVB rays.

SUN PROTECTION WITH TOPICAL ANTIOXIDANTS

Antioxidants also offer protection and prevent skin aging while nourishing and supplementing its deeper layers. They work by neutralizing dangerous free-radical molecules. Applying anti- oxidants topically, directly to the skin, is one way to address free-radical production, but not all antioxidant products con- tain adequate amounts of antioxidants to provide protection. Look for these ingredients, which are the most effective: vita- min C, vitamin E, ferulic acid, and phloretin.

Vitamin C is a water-soluble vitamin vital for producing collagen, which, as you know, gives skin its firmness and elasticity. It's also a powerhouse antioxidant that boosts the skin's radiance, prevents wrinkles, and is essential in cell proliferation. Vitamin C is also necessary for correcting skin pigmentation issues, reducing free radicals and facial redness. It regenerates vitamin E and provides protection from UVA and UVB rays.

Read labels carefully and look for a product that is pharmaceutical grade and tested for the highest quality and purity. The most common levels of vitamin C in topical products are 10, 15, or 20 percent. For people who have sensitive skin or have never used a vitamin C product before, 10 or 15 percent would be a good place to start. You must also assess what type of vitamin C is in the formula—it should be in the form of L-ascorbic acid, which is the only form of vitamin C that the body can effectively use.

Vitamin C is very unstable and degenerates when exposed to light and heat, and, unless it's properly processed and packaged in a dark glass bottle with a tight seal, it may oxidize before you have the opportunity to put it on your skin. Don't store it on a shelf that is exposed to any light or heat—your bathroom counter is not the best place. A vitamin C product that has turned yellow or brown has oxidized and should not be used.

Vitamin E is a well-known antioxidant with soothing, healing, and moisturizing properties. It is often used to help protect against sun damage and sunburn, to promote healing of burns and cuts, and to improve skin tone. It also prevents immuno-suppression and neutralizes free-radical damage.

Antioxidant properties of vitamin E have been well documented in many studies. In one study, when topical vitamin E was applied before exposure to cigarette smoke, the amount of free radicals produced was cut nearly in half as compared to skin not treated with vitamin E.[1]

Vitamin E needs to be in its pure or tocopherol form. Cosmetic companies will often use a different, less effective form in their products, which does not provide the benefits many consumers associate with vitamin E. A study published in the *Journal of the American Academy of Dermatology* found that topical vitamin C appears to provide superior protection from sun damage when used in conjunction with vitamin E.[2] As mentioned above, one reason that the two antioxidants work better when applied together is that vitamin C helps regenerate vitamin E.

Ferulic acid is an organic plant compound found in plant cell walls. It is a potent antioxidant and provides advanced protection from free-radical activity. When combined with vitamins C and E, ferulic acid reduces oxidative stress. With anti-inflammatory properties, it is effective in neutralizing free radicals. Research has also suggested that ferulic acid may help protect skin from UV damage, since it interferes with the process by which UV rays damage cell membranes.[3] In addition, ferulic acid helps prevent redness and sunburn from UVB rays.

Phloretin is a phenol (an aromatic organic compound) found in apple tree leaves and apricots. When combined with vitamin C and ferulic acid, it creates a potent antioxidant and provides advanced photo-aging protection. It also contributes to greater skin penetration of active ingredients in skin-care products for gradual release and delivery beneath the skin's surface.

While there are many different skin-care products that contain these ingredients, my favorite over-the-counter antioxidant skin-care product is the SkinCeuticals C E Ferulic, which is a combination antioxidant treatment with 15 percent L-ascorbic acid, 1 percent vitamin E, and 0.5 percent ferulic acid.

Topical Skin Care for Aging Skin

Over-the-counter skin creams or serums, whether cheap or expensive, can do four things and four things only: They can hydrate, exfoliate, even skin tone, or a combination of these things. If your skin is dry, a moisturizing cream can make it look more hydrated and feel smoother. If your skin is flaky, an exfoliating cream can rub off the flakes. If you have dull skin, pigmentation spots, or red patches, a lightening/brightening cream can improve your skin's appearance. And that's it. These products do not remove wrinkles. They do not get rid of eye bags. There is no such thing as a "facelift in a jar" or a "neck lift in a bottle" or a "laser in a serum." In other words, the actual signs of aging happening below the superficial levels of skin are completely unaffected by creams and serums.

Skin creams *do* work as intended, but only on a very superficial level. Anything you apply to the skin stays on the top, as the stratum corneum is a physical barrier to those deeper levels. But it is those deeper layers, unreachable by topical products, that age. Imagine an umbrella. If you pour water over your umbrella, it will become wet, but you will stay dry. Applying skin creams to the surface of your skin works in the same way.

There is one exception, but you cannot get it at Sephora. You can only get it with a prescription from a physician. It's called retinoic acid, or tretinoin, and it is often referred to by one of its brand names, Retin-A. Retinoic acid, which physically spurs more collagen production, is *the only topical product shown to actually penetrate down to deeper layers of the skin.*

I see hundreds of patients every year who tell me that they have drawers in their bathroom filled with dozens of different skin products promising dramatic effects that never panned out. When they come to me, they're fed up and are finally ready to try something that makes a noticeable difference. The thousands of dollars many people spend on useless creams and ointments could finance Retin-A (which is extremely inexpensive) and Botox treatments for many years. If you're someone who's already wasted a great deal of money on skin care, I'm sorry that you are only just reading this. The bottom line is that no skin cream, serum, gel, ointment, or lotion—no matter the type, no matter the cost, no matter if it contains peptides or amino acids or antioxidants or caffeine or even retinol—will *reverse* the signs of aging.

I know how easy it is to get sucked into marketing schemes and to continue buying the newest products from the latest celebrity spokesperson, dermatologist, or surgeon. But most consumers buy something and use it for a month or two, see no difference, or find that the product irritates their skin or causes breakouts, and they stop using it and move on to the next one. They are looking for a magic formula they want to believe exists.

Some people think their expensive products are working due to the placebo effect. If you gather a group of people and give them water described as an expensive serum, 30 percent of them will use it and report that they notice a positive effect. (On the other hand, of course, if you really love your skin-care products and get the results you want from them, there's no reason to stop using them!)

As we age, our skin does need more help. Rather than buy into the façade of the cosmetics industry, there are several easy and inexpensive daily steps you can take for optimal skin at any age: exfoliating (skin resurfacing), moisturizing, building deeper collagen layers, and evening skin tone and reducing hyperpigmentation.

EXFOLIATING

The topmost layer of dead skin cells serves a vital purpose by protecting your skin from the elements. But they are, after all, dead, and you need to get rid of them, since more and more are produced every day. Skin-cell turnover naturally slows down with age—you might have noticed this if your skin seems duller or less vital than before. A simple exfoliation will strip away the dead cells, leaving your skin looking fresher and more even.

There are two ways to exfoliate the skin, chemically (with alpha- and beta-hydroxy acids) and mechanically. Alpha- and beta-hydroxy acids (AHAs and BHAs) diminish fine lines and wrinkles by enhancing the shedding of the stratum corneum. The FDA has approved them as effective in reducing wrinkles, spots, and other signs of aging, including sun damage. The more commonly used AHAs include glycolic acid, ascorbic acid, and lactic acid. No wonder Cleopatra allegedly loved to take milk baths to add a certain glow to her legendary skin—she didn't know that milk contains lactic acid, only that it worked! Common BHAs include salicylic acid (an aspirin-like compound) and benzoic acid. Some claim that these compounds improve the quality of the elastin fibers and the collagen density in the dermis, thus reversing some of the skin's deeper damage and sagging.

The effectiveness of these chemical exfoliants depends mainly on the FDA-regulated concentration of AHAs and BHAs rather than accompanying inactive ingredients with scientific-sounding names. For example, when glycolic acid, one of the most popular AHAs, is prescribed by a physician, the concentration is between 20 and 30 percent, providing significant benefits. Over-the-counter preparations of glycolic acid, on the other hand, are usually at 5 percent concentration—less than one-fifth the concentration of AHAs found in preparations that physicians use. Be aware that most products with AHA concentrations below 8 percent barely work.

Microdermabrasion is a form of mechanical exfoliation that helps slough away the stratum corneum of the epidermis to help increase cell turnover and give skin a healthy glow. Deeper microdermabrasion requires specialized equipment only available at your doctor's office. These treatments can range from $150 to $250, becoming expensive after multiple sessions. There are other options for at-home exfoliation. However, you should avoid apricot scrubs for routine daily facial exfoliation, as they have larger sharp particles that can cause micro-tears to the skin and lead to premature aging. Instead, try using over-the-counter microdermabrasion devices that employ smaller and more delicate particles. These are often handheld devices similar to a microdermabrasion machine at the doctor's office, but they are not as aggressive and can be used every day. My favorite at-home microdermabrasion device is the Microderm GLO Diamond Microdermabrasion System by Nuvéderm.

MOISTURIZING

Once the skin is exfoliated, it should be moisturized. A moisturizer's sole function is to provide hydration, especially when skin is very dry. It can't remove wrinkles, but its texture can help to temporarily minimize their appearance.

There are many good over-the-counter moisturizers available in drugstores, department stores, and beauty stores such as Sephora. You do *not* need to see the doctor for a simple moisturizer or spend a ridiculous amount of money on one.

One of the least expensive everyday moisturizers that is available everywhere is Cetaphil. The Cetaphil Daily Hydrating Lotion is a moisturizing formula that is fast-acting, long-lasting, and helps hydrate extra-dry skin. It is nongreasy, nonirritating, noncomedogenic (doesn't cause pimples), and fragrance free. I recommend it for sensitive, allergenic, and acne-prone skin, and it can also be used safely on patients after surgery.

One of the most expensive moisturizers on the market is La Mer's Crème de la Mer, which I have found has wonderful moisturizing properties but literally costs twenty times more than a simple moisturizer like Cetaphil. Does this make it twenty times better? Not in my opinion, although I have many patients and even family members who swear by it. There are many, many other companies that sell proprietary moisturizers that are effective. As long as you use it daily, I think any moisturizer is good, as long as it hydrates your skin and is nongreasy, nonirritating, noncomedogenic, and fragrance free.

BUILDING DEEPER COLLAGEN LAYERS

Peptides, punicic acid, and vitamin A are the three topical agents that have been clinically proven to stimulate key constituents of the deeper dermal layers of the skin matrix: collagen, elastin, and glycosamnoglycans (GAGs).

Peptides are essentially chains of amino acids or proteins. Palmitoyl pentapeptide-4 is a skin-reparative and rejuvenation peptide found in a variety of topical products. Some companies, however, claim that the power of peptides in skin-care preparations can mimic the effects of Botox. This is not true, as no topical cream can penetrate into the facial muscles, which lie deep below the skin. Peptide products only work on the lines and wrinkles and *not* directly on the muscle activity.

Punicic acid is one of the main ingredients in pomegranate seed oil and is effective in cell regeneration and proliferation in the deeper dermis of the skin. Pomegranate seed oil is also effective in preventing skin cancer and is found to reduce lesions and tumors. Mainly known for its nourishing, moisturizing, and protective properties, pomegranate seed oil is increasingly being used in lip balms, face creams, lotions, and facial serums, as it has been found to soften dry, irritated, and aging skin. It activates the growth of keratinocytes (a major constituent of the epidermis) and is believed to play an important role in the synthesis of collagen. Overall, it helps to retain and improve skin elasticity, reducing the appearance of wrinkles and fine lines.

Cosmetic skin-care products use an extract of pomegranate seeds and combine it with other chemical ingredients. As a result, most of the seeds' properties are lost due to over-processing, making the products ineffective. Since many pomegranate seed products are also very expensive, the best solution is to make your own. Simply put a handful of pomegranate seeds in a blender to make juice, blend, strain, and apply directly on your skin or any affected area. Since no processing or artificial ingredients are involved, the seeds' properties remain intact. This might be a little messy, but it's worth a try.

Vitamin A was the first vitamin to be used topically for the treatment of damaged skin. The category of vitamin A derivatives includes retinol (vitamin A alcohol) and tretinoin (retinoic or vitamin A acid). These derivatives work by inducing a thickening of the epidermis, increasing the proliferation of skin cells, and as hormones to activate specific genes and proteins

Retinol Versus Retin-A

Do not confuse retinol with Retin-A, a brand name of retinoic acid/tretinoin. Retinol is a common and much-hyped ingredient in many over-the-counter products. It is very expensive but is only one one-hundredth the strength of retinoic acid. A tube of this highly diluted product can cost $300 to $400 per month—yet, remember, it is one one-hundredth as effective as a tube of Retin-A, which only costs about $50 and lasts for about three months.

Retinol is also very unstable and will degrade in the presence of light within minutes. That's why it is often sold in dark-colored jars: to help prevent dispersion of the molecules. Open the jar, put it on, and you've basically deactivated it.

Topical tretinoin was the original form of vitamin A that has been studied and proven to work, but it must be prescribed by a doctor. In randomized, prospective, placebo-controlled trials, tretinoin was definitively proven to reduce fine lines and wrinkling, roughness, and laxity. It is by far one of the best products you will ever use on your skin because it is so effective.

The key to success with Retin-A and other variations is that it should be used consistently, and it often isn't. The biggest problem is that consumers don't stick with its use because of the side effects. You can get badly sunburned when you use it, so sunscreen is a must. (This is actually a great side benefit, because it encourages the good habit of daily sunscreen use.) Retin-A can also cause irritation and drying at first. Start with a low concentration. If you can't tolerate daily use, you can use it every other day or every few days to avoid redness and flaking until your skin adjusts. Remember that Retin-A doesn't work overnight; results take about six months to appear.

If you want to try tretinoin, talk to your physician or dermatologist about a prescription for Retin-A. Follow the directions carefully and stick with it. Be patient. It will work—in fact, Retin-A is the *most important* cream to use to fight aging.

Be Wary of "Cosmeceuticals"

Cosmeceuticals are a marketer's dream. They are skin-care products that claim to have clinical strength and proven results, but these are not prescription-grade products. The active ingredients might be good, but they still have to be diluted to be sold without a prescription. You can almost always purchase a stronger and more effective skin-care product at a cheaper price from your doctor.

in the dermal layers. This hormonal activity increases deposits of new collagen in the dermis, reversing the thinning of this layer that occurs with age.

EVENING SKIN TONE AND REDUCING HYPERPIGMENTATION

Skin color is determined by the concentration of melanin—pigmentation produced by melanocytes—in the epidermis. Caucasians have the same number of melanocytes as Africans, but the melanin concentration in Africans is higher. Skin *tone* is classified by six different skin types, skin color, and reactions to sun exposure in the Fitzpatrick scale, developed in 1975 by dermatologist Thomas B. Fitzpatrick:

SKIN TYPE	SKIN COLOR	REACTION TO SUN EXPOSURE
Type I	Very white or freckled	Always burn
Type II	White	Usually burn
Type III	White to olive	Sometimes burn
Type IV	Brown	Rarely burn
Type V	Dark brown	Very rarely burn
Type VI	Black	Never burn

Uneven skin tone, including dark spots, freckles, white spots, or blotches, is very common. Hormone imbalance and sun exposure are the two most common causes. When skin gets lighter, it's called hypopigmentation; when it gets darker, it's called hyperpigmentation. People with Type III skin or greater on the Fitzpatrick scale are generally at a higher risk for pigment issues.

Because pigmentation spots and skin tone issues are so common, over-the-counter lightening creams that can treat them have been around for decades. The most popular bleaching ingredient in the United States is hydroquinone. It can, however, cause a skin discoloration called ochronosis, particularly in those with darker skin tones, that can leave users with blue-black areas, gray-brown spots, tiny yellow-to-brown bumps, or thickening skin. As a result, its use has been banned in Europe and other places around the world, but you can still buy lightening creams in the United States with up to a

2 percent concentration of hydroquinone. It's better to use a product with a 1 percent or lower concentration to avoid negative skin reactions.

Fortunately, newer skin lightening creams have been developed. Look for products containing kojic acid, disodium glycerophosphate, L-leucine, phenylethyl resorcinol, and undecylenoyl phenylalanine. Studies have shown them to be an effective alternative to hydroquinone.[4]

The Beauty Diet: Six Super Antioxidants and Nutrients for Aging Skin

When you don't eat right, your skin knows it and your skin shows it. Your color and tone will be off, making you look ashy or sallow. And, as mentioned previously, if there isn't enough fat in your diet, your skin can look haggard and drawn.

Many of my patients ask advice about the best things to eat and drink for their skin (and, of course, their overall health), and these suggestions are all extremely easy to incorporate into your lifestyle. You can use specific supplements or eat specific foods naturally containing micronutrients that are particularly nourishing for skin and circulation.

BEAUTY DIET SUPPLEMENTS

Even if you eat the most nutritionally balanced, organic, and plant-based diet, you may still not be ingesting as many nutrients as you think. This is often due to soil depletion and over-processing—and it's next to impossible for you to know what's been affecting your food chain unless you buy directly from farmers who tell you exactly how they grow and harvest their crops. One easy solution is to take high-quality, skin-supporting antioxidants in the form of daily supplements. You can also take a high-potency multivitamin that includes antioxidant-packed nutrients, as the effects of antioxidants are very synergistic; certain combinations can enhance the potency of each of the individual components. Or you can take individual supplements. This is what I recommend for the average adult:

ALPHA LIPOIC ACID

Alpha lipoic acid is a fat-soluble and water-soluble antioxidant/anti-inflammatory compound, which allows it to work inside and outside of your body's cells.

As a supplement: It may guard against a number of health conditions and also have anti-aging effects on your skin. The suggested dose of alpha lipoic acid for antioxidant support is approximately 40 mg/day.

In food: Dietary sources include organ meats, red meat, and brewer's yeast.

OMEGA-3 FATTY ACIDS

Omega-3 fatty acids are part of a group of essential fatty acids, particularly α-linolenic acid (ALA), eicosapentaenoic acid (EPA), and docosahexaenoic acid (DHA), which our bodies are unable to synthesize on their own, so we need to get them from outside sources. Omega 3s are an excellent anti-inflammatory efore be useful in treating a wide variety of skin conditions.

As a supplement: DHA and EPA are commonly found in fish oils. Fish oil has been shown to be an even more effective anti-inflammatory than aspirin and has no serious health side effects. The suggested dose is 3,000 mg/day.

In food: A good source for ALA is flaxseeds. Try to eat oily fish such as salmon and mackerel at least once or twice a week.

VITAMIN C (L-ASCORBIC ACID)

Vitamin C is the cofactor required to form new collagen in your skin.

As a supplement: The suggested dose is 1,000 mg/day.

In food: Vitamin C is found in citrus fruits and berries.

VITAMIN E

The primary role of vitamin E in the skin is to prevent damage induced by free radicals and reactive oxygen species; therefore, the use of vitamin E in the prevention of UV-induced damage has been extensively studied.

As a supplement: The suggested dose is 300 IU/day.

In food: Good sources of vitamin E are almonds, sunflower seeds, avocado, spinach, sweet potato, and wheat germ oil.

VITAMIN B5 (PANTOTHENIC ACID)

Vitamin B5 guards against a number of health conditions in addition to having anti-aging effects on your skin. A study on skin disorders found that topical vitamin B5 combats aging and acne by improving skin hydration, maintaining skin elasticity, and increasing skin softness.[5] The study also suggested that B5 has anti-inflammatory properties, making it useful in the treatment of skin scaling, roughness, dryness, and improvement of fine lines and wrinkles.

As a supplement: The suggested dosage of vitamin B5 for anti-inflammatory support is 50 to 100 mg/day.

In food: Good sources are chicken liver, sunflower seeds, egg yolk, broccoli, fish, and pomegranate.

POLYPHENOLS

Polyphenols are flavonoids found in a variety of foods, particularly green tea, that have been extensively studied for their potential health effects, including cardiovascular disease, hepatitis, and some cancers. Green tea has been shown to aid in the fight against sun damage by quenching free radicals and reducing inflammation, and it has also been shown to synergistically enhance SPF when used with sunscreen.

As a supplement: The suggested dosage is 1 cup of green tea each day.

In food: Polyphenols are also found in berries, red wine, olives, chocolate, grape skins and seeds, and walnuts.

In-Office Skin Resurfacing: Peels, Mechanical Exfoliation, Microneedling with PRP, IPL Therapy, and Lasers

Skin resurfacing is the term for procedures designed to improve the appearance of fine lines and wrinkles on your face. They range from superficial, to medium depth, to deep treatments. The difference between each has to do with the layer of skin they remove: Superficial treatments generally remove and resurface the epidermis, or top layer of the skin; medium-depth treatments get down to the medium depth (half-thickness) of the dermis; and deep treatments get down into the deeper two-thirds of the dermis. The deeper your wrinkles, the more aggressive you'll likely want your treatment to be, as it needs to penetrate into the deeper layers of skin.

You should not undergo any skin resurfacing treatments if you have a recent tan or sunburn or have taken Accutane (or any of the potent drugs containing isotretinoin, used to treat acne) for the past six months, as any of these can cause skin discoloration or scarring.

SUPERFICIAL TREATMENTS

These procedures are considered "lunchtime" treatments, since they don't take very long and don't leave you looking like you just got the worst sunburn of your life, so you can return to work after a treatment. They can result in some mild redness and irritation for a day or two but no raw surfaces to heal. There is generally little to no pain involved in these treatments, which are generally safe for patients with all skin types. Resurfacing treatments are usually performed repeatedly over a short period of time for maximum effect. For example, a superficial chemical peel with glycolic acid or microdermabrasion is done every few weeks for three months. Microdermabrasion, as mentioned previously, is a superficial treatment using a handheld device that sprays a stream of very fine crystals to exfoliate the skin. Repeated resurfacing will remove the dead layers of skin cells, tighten pores, and soften fine lines and wrinkles, but it will not stimulate collagen production in the deeper layers of skin and tighten the surface. Superficial resurfacing can't treat more substantial lines or wrinkles—especially lipstick-bleed lines, crow's feet, or deeper forehead lines—because these treatments don't penetrate deep enough into the skin. Microneedling penetrates through the skin surface and thus is more effective than microdermabrasion.

MICRONEEDLING WITH PRP

Skin-needling, also known as collagen induction therapy (CIT) or microneedling procedure, is a process that helps eliminate fine lines and wrinkles using your skin's natural abilities to heal itself and to produce collagen and elastin. The technique uses sterile tiny microneedles that create several controlled micro injuries to your skin. By doing so, the micro channels that are created initiate the repair process of the skin, naturally generating elastin and collagen that are ideal for smoothing your wrinkles, fine lines, acne scars, and traumatic scars. The micro channels created through this treatment provide direct pathways to your skin's deeper layers and allow for the maximum absorption of topical products, thus boosting their effects within the deeper skin layers.

One state-of-the-art skin topical is PRP, or platelet rich plasma. It is a concentration of platelets in the human blood crucial for wound healing. When it is used with microneedling, it releases crucial growth factors to speed up the repair process of your body and stimulate new elastin and collagen. The PRP is created from your own body: A small blood sample is extracted and the platelet plasma gets separated from the other elements by centrifuging the blood. It gets applied topically during and immediately after microneedling your skin.

The major benefit of combining PRP and microneedling is younger-looking skin with fewer signs of aging through the reduction of wrinkles and fine lines. Other benefits may include improvements to hypopigmentation, traumatic scars, and acne scars. Generally, microneedling with PRP creates a glow to the skin for a fresher appearance. All this is achieved without the heat trauma associated with lasers or other similar treatment devices. Because of the lack of heat energy, microneedling is suitable for all types of skin, including darker skin that is generally not suitable for laser therapy.

MEDIUM AND DEEP RESURFACING

Medium or deep resurfacing can be painful and take time to heal—but, of course, it will also last a lot longer. I also often do peels during facelift surgery, since my patients are already sedated or numbed. More time-effective, combining procedures means there is only one healing period. The most common acid used for these peels is trichloroacetic acid (TCA), in percentages of 20, 30, 35, and 40; the higher the number, the deeper the peel. At lower concentrations, the peel can be applied with the use of a local anesthetic to numb the skin.

After a TCA peel is applied, there is no more pain or burning. You'll need to apply moisturizing ointments for a week. After about four days, the dead skin surface peels off, almost like the way old paint flakes off a wall. By the end of the first week, all the old skin has peeled away, leaving very smooth, new pink skin (resembling a sunburn) underneath. You can use camouflaging makeup as soon as a week after the procedure, and the pinkness gradually fades over the following three weeks.

The most aggressive and deepest way to resurface the skin is with a phenol peel or macrodermabrasion. Since these procedures resurface to the deep dermal layer called the reticular dermis, they can remove the deepest wrinkles, causing the skin to tighten with the production of more collagen. Due to the aggressiveness of deep resurfacing, phenol peels carry greater risks of scarring and hypopigmentation, or skin lightening. The initial healing phase for these procedures is much longer, approximately two weeks, and the pink tone to the skin can last up to three months.

Phenol produces the most dramatic results and is the most effective peeling agent available. It produces a new zone of collagen that is thicker than that produced by laser or microdemabrasion. Phenol is absorbed through the skin, metabolized by the liver, and subsequently excreted by the kidneys.

However, the toxicity of phenol may be significant, and over-doses may injure these organs, leading to heart problems. For this reason, phenol peels should always be done by a physician who regularly performs them, in an operating room with a board-certified anesthesiologist present.

Unlike *micro*dermabrasion, *macro*dermabrasion is a much more aggressive treatment, similar to a medium or deep peel. While chemical peels use chemical energy, and laser resurfacing uses heat energy, dermabrasion is the process of mechanically removing the damaged layers of skin with a rotating brush or a diamond wheel—it's like using a sophisticated version of sand-paper. Because macrodermabrasion is extremely dependent on the skill of the surgeon, it can be viewed almost as an art, with the surgeon sculpting the skin. It works extremely well on deeper lines, especially the lipstick-bleed lines that radiate around the lips. The healing phase is usually two weeks. An occlusive dressing is worn during the healing process, as with laser resurfacing. The skin's surface also tends to weep, drain-ing fluid for the first few days, but this is a normal part of the post-procedure recovery.

IPL THERAPY

IPL stands for Intense Pulse Light Therapy, an energy-based system that sends out intense light of all wavelengths to interact with the skin in different ways. IPL treatments are non-ablative, meaning they do not melt the skin away with light and heat energy like their more aggressive counterparts, and they are *not* lasers, which makes them safer than, but not as effective as, some lasers. Still, IPL devices are considered skin-resurfacing workhorses because they treat many skin conditions with little or no healing downtime. They're a good option if you want a superficial treatment that will give your skin a more even tone and texture and expect only modest results after multiple sessions.

IPL is used to treat skin discoloration, brown or age spots, acne, rosacea, unwanted hair, and actinic keratosis, or pre-cancerous lesions. It's also often combined with other treatments such as Botox, microdermabrasion, and peels. Minor discomfort—comparable to a rubber band snapping on your skin—is typical for treatment with IPL. There are very few side effects, and IPL treatments require almost no healing time. Afterwards, dark spots may appear darker, and red spots may appear bruised, as they lift through the skin and migrate off.

Normally, IPL treatments are performed every three to six weeks, and a series of four to six treatments are recommended. Sometimes more treatments than expected are necessary, depending on how resistant the condition is—some patients may require up to eight or ten sessions. After full treatment, most people continue to need one or two treatments a year to prevent recurrence of their condition. When receiving IPL, it is imperative that patients avoid the sun and *always* use sunscreen—exposure to UV radiation will undo IPL's effects, wasting time and money.

LASERS

There are hundreds of lasers on the market today, and new types continue to launch all the time. A laser is a high-energy light beam that is extremely focused, capable of delivering high amounts of energy to a small area. Some lasers can specifically target a particular color or molecule to treat or remove it, and some can remove skin that is sun-damaged and wrinkled by vaporizing the damaged layers. Lasers of different frequencies and energy levels can treat a variety of skin problems, including unwanted hair, acne, port wine stains, scars, psoriasis, skin cancers, tattoos, blood vessels, wrinkles, laxity and sagging, freckles, scars, and stretch marks. To optimize any skin-resurfacing treatment, you may need a combination of several lasers.

LIGHT TOUCH LASERS

Light touch lasers (Nd:YAG, Alexandrite, and Pulsed Dye) are designed for superficial treatments. They are the gentlest, as they are non-ablative. Light touch lasers reorganize the collagen in the dermal layers of the skin, tighten it, and give it a better texture. A "cool touch" version is available when a cooling tip is used to minimize the patient's discomfort during treatment.

ABLATIVE LASERS

Unlike light touch lasers, ablative lasers remove layers by vaporizing or melting the skin. This encourages the growth of healthy new cells. They're the laser equivalent of a medium-depth chemical peel and are very effective at destroying unwanted tissue, but they require a week-long recuperation. The erbium YAG (Er:YAG) laser is most commonly used for fine lines and wrinkles, since it causes collagen contraction and new collagen formation in the dermal layers of the skin. It's less aggressive than a carbon dioxide (CO_2) laser and uses a different wavelength of light that results in less thermal injury.

The advantage to the Er:YAG laser over the CO_2 laser is a lower risk of scarring and lightening of skin tone, which is a common complaint from patients who receive these kinds of treatments. The thermal effect of the CO_2 laser on collagen causes the skin to tighten a little more than it would after a medium-depth peel. It's more effective on deeper wrinkles than the Er:YAG laser, since it removes damaged, aged skin, as well as heating the deeper skin layers to promote new collagen production. But with this effectiveness comes the increased risk of hypopigmentation and scarring. I recommend the Er:YAG laser to my patients with darker skin tones for this reason.

As with medium-depth chemical peels, all raw surfaces heal after seven days, though the skin remains pink for the next three weeks. Extensive treatment with the ablative CO_2 laser can mean two to three weeks of open skin wounds and weeping and crusting of the skin. This long recuperation makes it a less attractive option for most of my patients, and I prefer to use fractional lasers instead.

FRACTIONAL LASERS: THE EAST COAST LASER

Fractional lasers have a shorter healing time and fewer complications than the older versions of ablative lasers and are

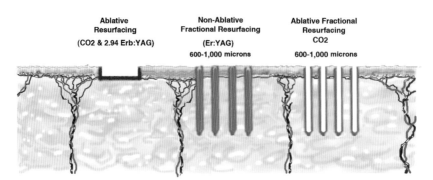

Figure 14: This diagram shows the progression of laser skin rejuvenation technology and the depth of penetration, from the older fully ablative CO_2 (left) to the newest fractional ablative lasers (right).

just as good at skin resurfacing, wrinkle removal, and facial rejuvenation. With this device, the laser beam is broken up, or fractionated, into many small micro-beams, separated so that when they strike the skin's surface, small areas of the skin between the beams are not hit by the laser, but left intact. These small areas, called micro-treatment zones, create new collagen to replace the collagen damaged by aging and sun exposure—which is what causes wrinkles. The new collagen produced by the laser injury "plumps" up the wrinkles (Figure 14).

Fractional lasers are a favorite of my Park Avenue patients. On average, they remove 60 to 70 percent of deeper lines and wrinkles, leaving a few character lines that make the face look natural and normal (Figure 15). Because of the fractionated nature of these lasers, the skin does not lose its color or become pale, waxy, or white, and there is essentially no risk of scarring. The intact skin between the micro-treatment zones allows for much more rapid healing, which makes them safer to use on darker skin. The Er:YAG fractional laser usually requires three

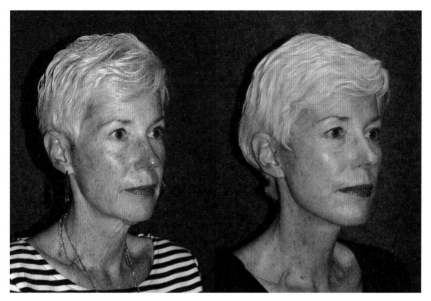

Figure 15: Before (left) and after (right) of a woman who had a fractional CO_2 laser for wrinkles and discoloration of her skin including hyperpigmentation (brown spots). This laser creates smooth, natural-appearing skin without making the skin look waxy or manipulated. She also had her jawline and neck lifted with a MADE facelift (see page 275).

The Danger of Too Many Chemical Peels

Have you ever noticed how the facial skin of older Hollywood celebrities can appear pale, almost translucent, yet line-free? Having too many deep peels in an attempt to try to erase every line on your face makes the skin look waxy. Many of my patients tell me they are afraid of this look: line free but artificial. While they want to reduce the number and severity of wrinkles on their faces, they also want to preserve some lines and creases so that they look as natural as possible. The best treatment to accomplish this is fractional laser resurfacing.

to five treatments to get good results and has a three- to five-day recovery time. Fractional CO_2 lasers go even deeper, requiring only one treatment, but often take one week to ten days to heal.

It's impossible to stress how important it is to take care of your skin. Healthy skin is beautiful skin and beautiful skin goes a long way in making you feel youthful and confident. Skin health should be the first stop on your plastic surgery journey. You may have other, unrelated concerns that facial plastic surgery can address, but if you are interested in maintaining your youthfulness, your skin should be a priority.

Now that we have demystified skin, the following chapter will delve into other nonsurgical options to address wrinkles, sagging skin, and other conditions most often related to aging.

---

1 Pravithra Rajagopalan et al., "How Does Chronic Cigarette Smoke Exposure Affect Human Skin? A Global Proteomics Study in Primary Human Keratinocytes," *OMICS* 20, no. 11 (2016), 615–626, doi: 10.1089/omi.2016.0123, https://www.ncbi.nlm.nih.gov/pubmed/27828771.

2 John C. Murray et al., "A Topical Antioxidant Solution Containing Vitamins C and E Stabilized by Ferulic Acid Provides Protection for Human Skin Against Damage Caused by Ultraviolet Irradiation," *Journal of the American Academy of Dermatology* 59, no. 3 (2008), 418–425, doi: 10.1016/j.jaad.2008.05.004, https://www.ncbi.nlm.nih.gov/pubmed/18603326.

3 Ibid.

4 Francesca Pintus et al., "New Insights into Highly Potent Tyrosinase Inhibitors Based on 3-heteroarylcoumarins: Anti-melanogenesis and Antioxidant Activities, and Computational Molecular Modeling Studies," *Bioorganic & Medicinal Chemistry* 25, no. 5 (2017), 1687–1695, doi: 10.1016/j.bmc.2017.01.037, https://www.ncbi.nlm.nih.gov/pubmed/28189394.

5 Gabriella Fabbrocini and Luigia Panariello, "Efficacy and Tolerability of a Topical Gel Containing 3% Hydrogen Peroxide, 1.5% Salicylic Acid and 4% D-panthenol in the Treatment of Mild-Moderate Acne," *Giornale Italiano di Dermatologia e Venereologia* 151, no. 3 (2016), 287–291, https://www.ncbi.nlm.nih.gov/pubmed/26761768.

5

Nonsurgical Facial Rejuvenation with Injectable Treatments

Over the last two decades, there has been a remarkable shift in how skilled doctors, dermatologists, ophthalmologists, and plastic surgeons tackle aging concerns *without* surgery. Now, not only are there dozens more devices and products to smooth out wrinkles and make your skin brighter and more vibrant, injectable fillers can replace lost volume and Botox can erase wrinkles. If you're interested in procedures that will effectively rejuvenate and refresh your face, but you aren't yet ready for surgery, this chapter will give you an overview of the most popular noninvasive injectable treatments available today.

Injectable Fillers

TEMPORARY HYALURONIC ACID FILLERS (JUVEDERM, RESTYLANE, BELOTERO)

Hyaluronic acid is a sugar-based gel injected into the skin to diminish folds and wrinkles—the most common being the marionette lines running from the edges of the lips down to the chin, the lipstick-bleed lines, and the nasolabial folds (the smile lines that run between the nose and mouth). Hyaluronic acid is found naturally in our skin, bones, and cartilage, and what doctors use for injections is bioengineered in a lab, so there is no need for skin testing. It is a safe compound that degrades gradually in your body over time. These fillers can also be used to add volume to thin lips, flat cheeks, and weak chins. As our faces lose volume and descend with age, adding filler can help lift cheeks and support jawlines and jowls. It can also be used to fill dark under-eye circles (Figure 16).

One of the most common questions patients ask me is, "What's the best filler?" Juvederm and Restylane are the two most popular dermal fillers in the United States (there are also more than a hundred fillers derived from different formulations of hyaluronic acid gels available in Europe), but the answer is that there is no universally "best" filler. It just depends on what you are trying to correct. Hyaluronic acid fillers have different consistencies, called G Prime. Those with a low G Prime are thin, like pancake syrup, and are great to combat smile lines and folds. Juvederm Ultra is a low G Prime filler that is best for this purpose. Other fillers have a high G Prime—their

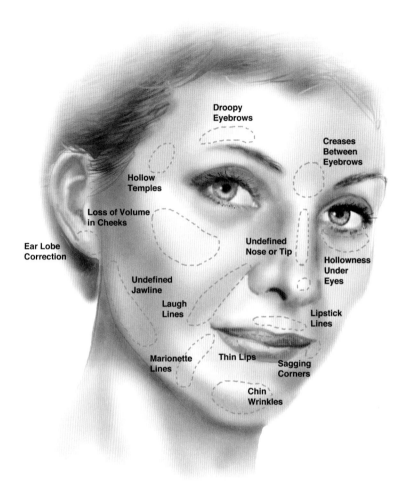

Figure 16: Sites where the face can be rejuvenated with facial fillers: Eyes, jawlines, and smile lines can be smoothed, and cheeks, chins, and noses can be reshaped without surgery, just to name a few examples.

consistencies are like gelatin, so they are bouncy and support-ive. They are best used to fill chins and cheeks and lift jowls. Restylane Lyft and Voluma are both high G Prime fillers.

On average, Restylane and Juvederm last for six months to one year, while Belotero lasts for six months or less, and

Voluma has been shown to last up to two years in FDA trials. Juvederm is generally not used around the eyes, as the material tends to absorb water, which can make your eyes look puffy; Restylane and Belotero are a better choice around the eyes.

Restylane has developed a product called Restylane Lyft, with larger hyaluronic gel particles that allow it to lift as well as fill the areas of injection. It's often used to restore lost volume in cheeks, on the sides of the chin where jowls start to form, and in the marionette lines.

TEMPORARY NON-HYALURONIC ACID FILLERS (RADIESSE, SCULPTRA)

This category of fillers has the additional ability to stimulate new collagen over time. These fillers should never be injected into the lips or around the eyes because they can also cause nodules to form. Radiesse is made from the same mineral substance as our bones and consists of microscopic calcium particles suspended in a water-based gel. This is also a very safe material used for dental reconstruction, bone growth, and vocal cord injection, and, like hyaluronic acid, it gradually degrades harmlessly in the body. Radiesse usually lasts between twelve and eighteen months. It is used in the deepest of facial folds due to its more viscous nature and can't be injected in the superficial skin layers, since it has a white color that shows through.

I often use Radiesse to augment the nasolabial folds, lift corners of the mouth, and contour the cheeks, chin, and jawline. It works well in heavier, droopier faces, especially in the

Reversing Injectable Fillers

One of the main benefits of hyaluronic acid fillers is that they can be easily reversed if you don't like the results (if too much was injected or if the area feels lumpy). An enzyme called hyaluronidase (or Vitrase) can be injected into the affected area, which literally eats up the hyaluronic acid within twenty-four to forty-eight hours. Patients often come to me to dissolve away poorly executed fillers, and sometimes more than one treatment is needed to remove all the material injected. You can then reinject the area with more precision after one week.

cheeks or other areas of the face, as it's more supportive than hyaluronic acid. I do not use Radiesse as much as I did years ago because Voluma and Restylane Lyft are good alternatives and can be reversed. If you do not like your Radiesse treatment, you have to wait for the material to naturally dissolve away, which, as mentioned, can take up to eighteen months.

Sculptra is composed of poly-L-lactic acid, a biodegradable polymer used in suture material. It is a safe biocompatible material injected below the surface of the skin, primarily in areas of fat loss. Sculptra is actually not a wrinkle filler but a bio-activator, or "volumizer," that works by stimulating the body to produce new collagen at injection sites, replacing lost volume and contours to restore a fuller, more youthful appearance. Sculptra should not be used for more superficial lines and folds because it causes nodules that will persist for many

What Is a Liquid Facelift?

Many people who are apprehensive about or just don't want surgery often ask me about a "liquid facelift," which is just a fancy term for using fillers to help lift drooping portions of the face, usually the cheeks, jowls, and jawline. A liquid facelift works best in patients who are in their forties to sixties. The best fillers in this situation are fillers like Voluma or Restylane Lyft. They are usually injected deeply on top of the bones of the cheek or jaw so they help support and lift the face (Figure 17).

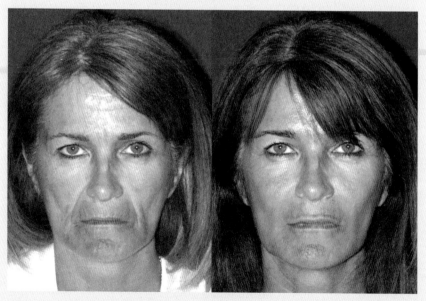

Figure 17: Before (left) and after (right) of a woman who had a nonsurgical "liquid facelift." Hyaluronic acid fillers were used to lift the cheeks, add volume to the face, and reduce the folds around the lower face and mouth. Her lips were filled to augment them and reduce lipstick-bleed lines. She also had Botox injected between her eyebrows to reduce the appearance of vertical wrinkles referred to as the "elevens."

months. Typically, you'll need two or three treatments with Sculptra to get the desired effect, so it will require more visits to get the desired outcome compared to traditional fillers, but it can last up to two years. One disadvantage that I have found with patients treated with Sculptra, and a reason that I prefer not to use it, is that when they have a facelift or other facial plastic surgery in the area previously injected, there is scar tissue that makes the operation more difficult.

TEMPORARY FILLERS ARE GREAT—UNTIL THEY AREN'T

Fillers work beautifully when they're injected by a doctor with a deft hand, a practiced eye, and a detailed knowledge of facial anatomy. When used in the right places on the right faces, they can give you nearly instantaneous results, smoothing skin by replacing lost volume, and making you look refreshed.

When overdone, on the other hand, they leave faces looking fake, puffy, and distorted. I am alarmed whenever I see women in their twenties, thirties, and forties who have overfilled cheeks. It may photograph well for a selfie, but in person it makes the face look monkey-like.

Because my patients are fearful of overfilling, I inject smaller amounts of filler at the upper parts of the cheek, and not lower down, where it distorts the face. I almost never inject more than one vial of filler (which is 1 milliliter of material) at one time. I have treated many patients for overfilled cheeks who have had six or more vials injected into their faces in just one session! I intentionally undertreat the area, let it settle, and add more filler one week later. By working slowly, the transformation is more gradual and natural contours can be preserved. Less is more in this situation. What's worse is that overfilling the face actually can *make you age more rapidly.* Injecting filler into your face at a young age, and/or injecting too much of it, distends the tissues in your face, stretching them out and creating more skin, making a facelift necessary much sooner.

As we age, our facial skin becomes laxer, requiring an increasing amount of injectable material to lift what is drooping. This need is more common in the mid- to late forties and into the fifties. The problem is that the filler will actually weigh the face down, making it look unnaturally wide. Tightening becomes necessary to reposition what has fallen. Interestingly, patients don't realize that, in the long run, one facelift is likely to be less expensive than multiple noninvasive treatments. A decade of injectables and lasers can often cost two to three times more than surgery. It is not uncommon for patients to spend $7,000 to $8,000 on fillers in just two to three years.

WHEN TEMPORARY FILLERS GO WRONG AND HOW TO FIX THEM

Too much filler in too many places can leave people looking plastic, distorted, or even a lot older than intended. Unnatural firmness or lumps can occur anywhere fillers are injected, usually when too much filler is injected into one spot or too superficially (too shallowly) in the skin. The "Tyndall effect" is a discoloration that can appear if hyaluronic acid fillers are injected too superficially into the skin. It causes light to reflect through the skin, giving it a bluish tint. This discoloration occurs most commonly with eyelid injections to fill dark circles. Restylane and Belotero have a lower propensity to this discoloration. These problems can be dissolved away as described earlier, but with Radiesse or Sculptra, which are not hyaluronic acid fillers and can't be dissolved away, your only option is to attempt to camouflage uneven or irregular areas with an HA filler.

While rare, infections from injectable fillers can develop. These infections are called biofilms and present as persistent redness in the skin for weeks. Biofilms, which can persist and be antibiotic-resistant, can form even when you receive perfectly appropriate filler from an expert physician injector. If you notice any symptoms of infection, it is important to see your doctor immediately so that you can get treated with oral antibiotics.

PERMANENT FILLERS (ARTEFILL, COLLAGEN, SILICONE)

Permanent fillers sound like such a great idea: One visit to the doctor's office and you're done. But in reality, the possibility of a botched outcome with permanent fillers—with the only solution to reverse being surgery—far outweighs the benefits of convenience and cost. Because temporary fillers are so much easier to use and control, and because they wear off (and hyaluronic acid can be undone), I rarely use permanent fillers, although some of my colleagues do.

The only FDA-approved permanent filler for use in the face is Artefill, a mixture of synthetic beads and bovine collagen. After the collagen reabsorbs, the synthetic microspheres stimulate the body to generate its own natural collagen to encapsulate each individual microsphere, which fills up the wrinkles. An allergy test is usually done a month before treatment to make sure you're not allergic to the collagen.

The most commonly injected permanent facial filler in America is liquid silicone. Silicone is FDA-approved only for the treatment of detached retinas, so using it as a filler is considered off-label use—meaning it hasn't been specifically FDA-approved for that purpose, though it isn't technically illegal. (In fact, liquid silicone is used as a lubricant for hypodermic needles, so it's technically being introduced in tiny amounts every time anyone receives an injection of any kind, but it's such a miniscule amount it won't affect skin.) Silicone draws polarized reactions from both the public and physicians. While many doctors consider silicone too risky for facial cosmetic injections, it can be administered safely if injected by an experienced professional who uses an appropriate, medical injecting-grade silicone.

WHEN PERMANENT FILLERS GO WRONG AND HOW TO FIX THEM

As I mentioned in Chapter 3, take a look at Priscilla Presley over the years to see what can happen when a quack injects nonmedical-grade silicone into the face of an iconic, beautiful woman.

All permanent facial filler injections have three major risks that can't be easily reversed: over-injection, granulomas, and migration. The most notable complication is over-injection, which can leave patients with distorted features such as rounded faces, swollen cheeks, or misshapen and overly large lips. What can't be controlled by any physician, no matter how expert he or she is, is that a small percentage (1 to 3 percent) of patients will develop a chronic reaction to the filler, forming nodules called granulomas, or the filler can migrate away from wherever it was injected. Steroid injections can be used to try to reduce the granulomas, but this fails more often than not. Migration usually doesn't happen right away, but after many years (ten years or more), as facial tissues loosen and thin out, the filler can suddenly begin to show through the skin.

The only way to correct any of these problems is to surgically remove the filler, which can leave scars on a patient's face. This is why I prefer not to use permanent fillers. I also perform a lot of revision surgery on patients who've had complications from permanent filler injections, which has made me even more reluctant to use them.

Fat Transfer/Stem Cell Facelift

Another popular procedure is fat transfer, often referred to as a stem cell facelift. A stem cell facelift is a misnomer, as it is not a surgical procedure, nor does it actually lift the face. It's a procedure that uses fat suctioned from one area of the body transferred back into the areas of your face that need plumping. Since your own cells are used, there's no worry about the possibility of experiencing any reactions to them as you might with synthetic fillers.

What differentiates a stem cell facelift from the older fat transfer procedure is that the fat is harvested and injected with special cannulas to ensure the fat survives. Fat cells are extremely fragile, and the main goal is to make sure they survive once transplanted. Fat can be added back to the cheeks, jawline, smile and marionette lines, and to any deep circles under the eyes, creating the appearance of a lower eyelid lift without surgery (Figure 18). Fat is globular and thick and cannot be injected into fine surface lines, which would make them look lumpy.

The procedure itself is usually done on an outpatient basis. The fat is harvested from either the abdomen or the buttocks while the patient is under local anesthesia, using suction and aspiration with a needle. It's then processed to maximize the

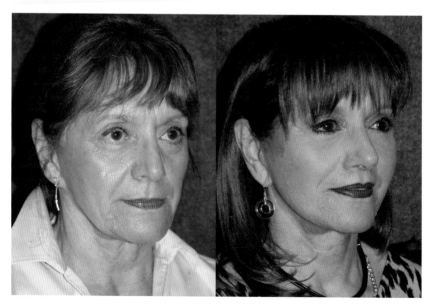

Figure 18: Before (left) and after (right) of a woman who underwent a stem cell facelift to lift her cheeks, fill the hollows under her eyes, and smooth her smile lines. Aging creates volume loss in the face, and replacing it with your own body fat and stem cells can create a long-lasting and natural-appearing result. She also had her jawline and neck lifted with a MADE facelift (see page 275).

stem cells in preparation for injection, and finally injected (again, while the patient is under local anesthesia) into the desired areas of the face.

Recovery takes about a week. There might be some initial bruising, swelling, and tenderness at the injection sites, which can be easily covered by makeup. The results typically last for three to five years. If you are very thin, with minimal body fat, you may not be a good candidate for fat transfer, as there won't be enough fat to harvest. If this is the case, I use the temporary fillers described earlier in this chapter instead.

Be aware that adult-derived stem cells found in your fat are not the same thing as the stem cells found in the umbilical cords of newborns, which can be stored for potential use in treating blood disorders and immune deficiencies. There is little research on further uses of adult stem cells, though, allegedly, the stem cells found in fat are meant to be a source for producing other hormone-like substances and growth factors to enhance both skin quality and the underlying fatty tissues.

One disadvantage of the stem cell facelift is the unpredictability of its effectiveness. I've found that a third of the time all of the fat remains in place after it's injected, a third of the time only part of it stays, and a third of the time none of it stays. There's simply no way to know in advance how well the procedure will work. If your fat doesn't take, you can try a secondary fat transfer. In my experience, as well as in the medical literature, it's reasonable to estimate that 30 percent of patients will need a second session to achieve their aesthetic goals, if not more. In that case, enough fat has usually been removed during the initial procedure and stored, so you'd only need to repeat the injections and not the harvesting.

WHEN FAT TRANSFER/STEM CELL FACELIFTS GO WRONG AND HOW TO FIX THEM

Like all procedures, facial fat transfers have their pros and cons. Because using fat as filler is unpredictable, most doctors err on the side of overfilling rather than underfilling, based on the assumption that, in most cases, a lot of the fat will be absorbed into the body. The risk of overcorrecting is the possibility that all of the fat does stay when injected, in which case the patient is going to be very, very unhappy with the results. He or she will look bloated and can even become afflicted with lumps and bumps. The only way to fix this is with corrective surgery, such as a facelift, to remove some of the fat, but it is very tricky to get the contours to look completely normal. Once again, less is more.

Most doctors won't tell you that body fat is hormonally active. It doesn't act like facial fat. It can grow if you gain weight. I know patients who had fat grafting, then put on twenty pounds and saw their faces become distorted. If your weight tends to yo-yo, it is best to use temporary fillers. Another problem may arise as a woman becomes post-menopausal and her metabolism and hormone levels are altered, which can cause the fat cells to enlarge, making it difficult to maintain her weight. The face can change shape years after a patient has had fat injections. I've seen many women in consultation who loved the results from their fat grafting for many years during their forties, but, when they hit their mid- to late-fifties, their

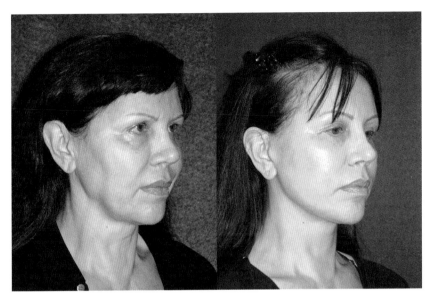

Figure 19: Before (left) and after (right) of a woman in her fifties who underwent a MADE facelift (described in Chapter 11). She had had a fat transfer a decade earlier and loved the result in her forties, but the fat grew with age, causing her face to look overly full and accelerated facial drooping. Using the MADE facelift technique, I reduced the excess fat and elevated her cheeks that were dragged down by the heaviness of the fat graft, re-creating a heart-shaped face.

faces suddenly started to look bloated. Worse, this happens at the same time that facial skin is starting to loosen due to the normal aging process, coupled with gravity. In other words, the fat grows and alters your face shape right when your facial skin is beginning to droop. Because of the unpredictability of this procedure, I recommend that women in their forties use less fat grafting in their faces and top off any additional volume correction with temporary fillers (Figure 19).

Injectable Fat Dissolver: Kybella

Kybella is a substance that breaks down fat cells, which your body then naturally excretes. It was created to treat excessive fullness and localized fatty tissue underneath the chin, and it's an excellent example of how marketing can create buzz around a product that often can't live up to the hype.

Kybella is advertised as an injection that is noninvasive (which is true) and will get rid of your double chin (which is only sometimes true). Most people will see the ad and think, "Great—just one little shot with no recovery time and I can kiss my turkey neck goodbye." These injections need to be repeated three or four times, spaced four to six weeks apart, for the best results. Kybella consists of bile acids that literally digest the fat under your neck—your neck blows up like a bullfrog for three to five days following each injection.

While the results can be good if you just have extra neck fat, the results are often disappointing for those with lax or drooping skin. Drooping neck skin can actually get worse when you deflate the fat, causing the skin to hang, similar to the way abdominal skin hangs after massive weight loss. Kybella only removes fat, not skin.

Surgical liposuction is a good alternative to Kybella for those with isolated fat deposits under the neck. Compared to Kybella's three or four separate treatments, and a cumulative fifteen to twenty days of swelling and recovery, one liposuction procedure on the same area has about a five-day recovery (see Chapter 10 for more details on liposuction).

To be fair, Kybella can work extremely well on younger patients whose skin still has a lot of elasticity and easily snaps back. For those who commit to all four sessions and who don't expect immediate results, it's possible to start to see a lot of improvement after the second session, as the body needs at least four to eight weeks to be able to break down the targeted fat cells. Unlike surgery, there is little risk for complications or scarring, and the most common side effects (mild redness at the treatment site, bleeding, bruising, and temporary numbness) normally go away within a day or two—but the swelling, as I said, can last up to five days after each session. The results are also permanent, as once the fat cells break down, they cannot reform.

Injectable Wrinkle Relaxers: Botox, Dysport, and Xeomin

What causes wrinkles? They're the result of the delicate facial muscles underneath your skin's surface contracting during normal daily use. In other words, over time, the skin covering the areas where you are naturally the most animated and expressive will begin to crease. That's why we tend to show wrinkles, lines, and folds around the eyes (crow's feet), between the eyes (elevens, or the glabellar lines), on the forehead (frown lines from concentration or anger), and around the mouth (smile lines, lipstick-bleed lines) (Figure 17).

Botox is made from highly purified and extremely dilute botulinum toxin (it cannot poison you—something patients worried about when it first came on the market). It works by blocking the nerve impulses to the wrinkle-producing muscles so that they don't contract, leaving the overlying skin smooth and unwrinkled. Of all the injectables that I offer, Botox is by

Don't Price-Shop for Botox

It's common to see ads (including Groupon offers) for Botox touting pricing far less expensive than the quote given to you by an experienced cosmetic dermatologist or plastic surgeon. There are two reasons for this. One is that Botox can easily be diluted. The more dilute it is, the shorter it lasts. So, you might end up paying a lot more if your injections wear off quickly.

The second is that any licensed physician, not only a specialized facial plastic surgeon, can legally give you injections. But do you really want your endocrinologist or gynecologist doing your Botox (or filler)? Would you want me to treat your diabetes or deliver your baby? I *could*, but I certainly wouldn't be the best doctor to do so. As you have read in this chapter, the risk of complications in these situations dramatically increases if you don't see someone with extensive training and experience in the specific procedure you are seeking.

far the most common and the most effective. I administer very precise injections into the areas selected for treatment, and any untreated muscles will continue to move as they always have.

Botox injections usually cause minimal discomfort, as the needle is very fine. The procedure is fairly quick—I've had patients come in for Botox during their lunch hour. It takes forty-eight to seventy-two hours before the effect is visible, and full penetration can take up to one week. Sometimes a touch-up may be necessary to even out the results at one week post-treatment. Patients often ask whether they will feel frozen after the injections, but Botox doesn't change how your skin feels—it just stops the muscles from moving. You'll still be able to laugh, smile, or frown, but without the resulting wrinkles.

It is absolutely not addictive in any way. I often make the comparison to hair color treatments. When you start to see your roots come back, you get a touch-up; when your wrinkles come back, you get a Botox touch-up if you want one (if you don't, your wrinkles will gradually reappear). Botox has been used for more than two decades to treat muscular disorders and is extremely safe. Complications are quite rare, unless the treatment is improperly administered or too much is used in the wrong place.

The downside to Botox is that it wears off after four to six months. I've found that if you get Botox over a regular period of time, it lasts longer than if you just get it once and then come back again a year or two later.

Botox can also be used to lift the eyebrows and the marionette lines, to relax the cords in the neck, and in other areas you can see in the Off-Label Botox Use sidebar on page 124. The best way to understand how Botox works is by understanding that there is a constant tug-of-war going on in any section of the face. There are muscles that lift a portion of the face (such as the eyebrows) and opposing muscles that pull it down. When Botox is injected into the muscle that pulls things down, the muscle that lifts wins, resulting in that portion of the face being elevated.

Off-Label Botox Use

Botox is intended to be used as a wrinkle relaxer (according to the product's label), but it can also be used in the following treatments:

Neck bands and cords: Botox can soften these cords if they are too prominent or look ropey.

Brow lift: This isn't the same as injecting Botox between the eyes or in the middle of the forehead. Instead, Botox is injected, using a different, specific method, near the eyebrows, to lift them up (Figure 20).

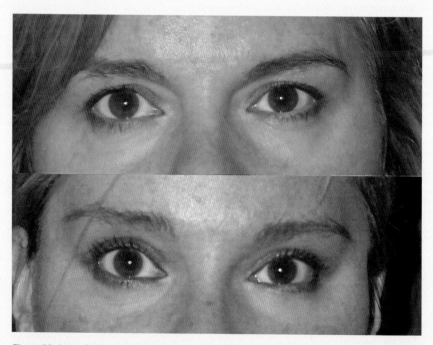

Figure 20: Before (top) and after (bottom) of a woman who had a "Botox brow lift." Botulinum toxin was used to lift the brows and open the eyes.

Drooping corner of the mouth: When injected near the corner of lips that turn downward (making you look like you're frowning when you actually aren't), it can lift the lips up and make you look happier.

Drooping tip of the nose: Sometimes, a droopy tip of the nose can be caused by an overactive muscle rather than by the nose cartilage itself. Botox can be injected between the nostrils to release this muscle and cause the tip to upturn slightly.

Gummy smile: If your gums look too exposed when you're smiling, Botox injections around the mouth can prevent your lips from elevating too much.

Pore size: Botox can even help those with acne and enlarged pores—injections just under the skin can diminish oil production in the sebaceous glands.

Other brands of the botulinum toxin are Dysport and Xeomin. Dysport acts more quickly, usually within twenty-four hours, so it might be a desirable option before a big social event or meeting. It lasts as long as Botox.

WHEN INJECTABLE WRINKLE RELAXERS GO WRONG AND HOW TO FIX THEM

Many patients are fearful of looking frozen or odd after they get Botox, and with good reason. They see Hollywood stars of a certain age whose foreheads are unnaturally smooth. But this happens even to "regular people" all over America, who have that same artificial, waxen sheen. This is one sign of too much Botox. It's actually not so much that the skin gets shiny, it's just that the smoothness created by Botox doesn't reflect light the way normally animated foreheads do; the skin looks shiny because it's become perfectly flat.

When too much Botox is placed in the horizontal forehead lines, it becomes impossible to lift the eyebrows. This can make you look frozen, like so many newscasters who appear expressionless even when their voices are animated. It may be tempting for television and film personalities and performers to overdo Botox, since they are shot in high definition, magnifying every wrinkle and line. But too much Botox can also cause your eyebrows to fall over your eyelids, making them look droopy. There is no way to fix this problem; it usually takes four to six weeks for the injections to wear off to the point where your eyes are not as droopy but the forehead lines are still corrected.

My patients want to maintain motion in their face and de-emphasize lines. I usually use half the normal dose of Botox to make sure the muscles around the eyebrows and eyelids still function, which softens the appearance and looks completely natural.

Botox can also cause a problem commonly referred to as "Spock eye." This is the result of injections made only in the center of the forehead, which creates a pronounced arch in the brow—like the look sported by Spock on *Star Trek* (Jack Nicholson's brows make this shape naturally). This can be corrected by injecting a small amount of Botox above the area where the eyebrows lift.

Botox injections around your eyes or eyebrows can migrate into the upper eyelid and cause it to droop, causing you to look as if you've had a stroke. This is a fairly rare condition called blepharoptosis and usually occurs when someone without a lot of experience administers the injections. The only remedy is to use eye drops called Iodipine that will make the eye open, but they only work for an hour or two at a time. The problem usually improves after six weeks, as the effects of the Botox start to wear off.

Injectables are so popular in part because they seem innocuous and low maintenance, but they can be as dangerous as any procedure that requires going under the knife. With knowledge and preparation come safety and success. Now that you know the basics, you can turn to any of the chapters in Part III for more precise details about which facial rejuvenation procedure is best for you.

PART
III

FINDING THE
SURGICAL PROCEDURE
THAT IS RIGHT FOR YOU

Please note that in this part of the book I have included specific sections on how procedures might differ depending on a patient's ethnicity and gender. Unless specified to the contrary, the information you'll read is applicable to all ethnicities.

6 Open Your Eyes

When my patients reach their forties and fifties, they often focus on the changes they see occurring around their eyes. At this age, their family, friends, and coworkers might start saying things like, "You look tired," or "You are working too hard; maybe you need some rest." To the frustration of many of my patients, no matter how young and energetic they may feel, their aging eyes suggest the exact opposite. Some changes, such as hanging eyelid skin and lower eyelid bags, are so dramatic that they can even impair vision.

One out of every three procedures I do is to rejuvenate the eyes. Even though these procedures are fairly routine, my patients are often incredibly apprehensive about them—and with good reason. Plastic surgery on the eye area carries the *most risk* for changing what is familiar about your face (and not in a good way). When botched, eye procedures can leave people with eyes so wide open, with brows so lifted, that they appear constantly startled, like a deer in headlights. My patients are worried about getting "cat eyes" or looking like Jocelyn Wildenstein, who is commonly referred to as the "cat woman." It is certainly possible to repair drooping eyes and foreheads, dark circles, and puffiness under your eyes effectively and naturalistically. The first step is to choose an experienced surgeon (as outlined in Chapter 3).

This chapter will describe procedures for eyes and for foreheads/brows, tailored to your needs and desired outcome, discussed in order of least to most invasive. Your eyes are the first thing people notice when they meet you. You don't want them to make you look old, but neither do you want to radically change your most prominent feature with a botched procedure. This chapter will help you avoid both.

What Happens to Your Eyes as You Age

As you learned in Part II, as we age, our skin loses its elasticity and begins to sag. This loss of elasticity, plus the development of fat deposits, causes a buildup of excessive skin on the upper and lower eyelids, as well as wrinkling. In addition, over time, our eyelid proportions change. The forehead drops, leading the eyebrows to droop over the eyes. In turn, the upper eyelid shortens, which is why it can become more difficult to apply makeup to the upper eyelids as we age. The sagging skin gets in the way, and what makeup is successfully deposited often disappears quickly during normal blinking. This excessive drooping of the upper eyelids is known as "hooding."

Drooping upper eyelids can also affect your vision, the correction of which is a medical, not a cosmetic, procedure, called a functional blepharoplasty (and therefore usually covered by insurance). Patients with this condition often suffer from discomfort in their foreheads caused by the overuse of muscles that are constantly strained to lift the sagging eyelids; they may also develop eyelid irritation due to the rubbing together of the excess folds of skin. The lower eyelids age differently. The fat under the eyes grows, creating bags and puffiness. At the same time, dark circles develop under these bags (called the tear trough, because they create a hollowed-out area). This is the result of volume loss along the cheekbones and the drooping of the cheeks. In other words, the upper eyelid becomes shorter while the lower eyelid becomes longer, a non-youthful combination.

There is also a strong genetic component to how your eyelids age. Patients often tell me that they started noticing the changes when they were in their twenties and that everyone in their family has the same issue. Unlike facelifts, I've done many eyelid procedures on women in their thirties because of this genetic predisposition.

Nonsurgical Eyelid Lifts

For a nonsurgical eyelid lift, I use different injectables to reestablish youthful proportions and to rejuvenate tired eyes—usually a reshaping combination of Botox and temporary fillers. This is less expensive than a liquid facelift because the area around the eye is smaller and requires fewer vials of material. Many patients start with this treatment in their thirties when they first notice changes. During their fifties, eye tissues become loose and droopy enough that injections lose their effectiveness, and this is when patients usually opt for eyelid lifts or brow lifts.

For upper eyelid correction, Botox is injected into the muscles that pull down the eyebrows. The injection sites are between the eyebrows and under the outer corner of the brows. Injecting these muscles with Botox releases them, allowing them to elevate, which makes the upper eyelids lift and the skin look less droopy. A great use to lift the eyelids by 2 to 3 millimeters, the treatment's only downside is that it lasts for just four to six months, requiring repeat injections two to three times a year, which can become costly over the long haul.

Correcting lower eyelids requires filling the hollowing effect under the eyes with a hyaluronic acid filler. The two safest fillers for this are Restylane and Belotero, because other fillers will either result in discoloration of the skin or draw water into the under-eye hollow from elsewhere in the body, causing puffy areas to appear along the cheeks. Using fillers to plump up the area under the lower lids will shorten the length of the lower eyelids and the distance from the lower eyelashes to the cheek, and reduce dark circles or sunken areas. This method can hide the smaller bags that form under the eyes (Figure 21). What's great about this procedure is that the filler under the eyes often lasts for one to one and a half years, which means you'll spend less on repeat treatments. For most patients, only

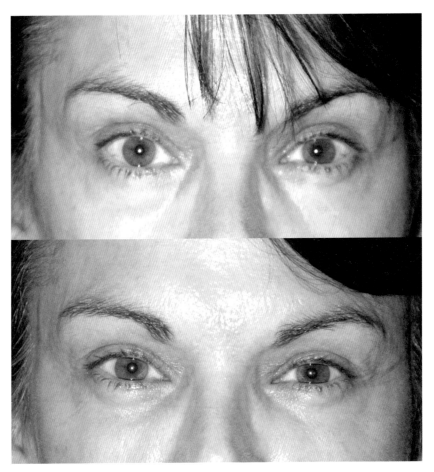

Figure 21: Before (top) and after (bottom) of a nonsurgical eyelift using hyaluronic acid filler. The filler is injected to fill the dark circles under the eyes and reduce the appearance of lower eyelid bags.

one vial of filler is required, split between two sides, so the procedure is also more affordable. If you have larger under-eye bags, this approach will not, unfortunately, improve them sufficiently, and a lower eyelift may be necessary, instead.

Filler Fatigue

Many of my patients develop what I call "filler fatigue"—they become tired of coming back again and again for filler injections and wary of the escalating expense. In these cases, we will perform fat transfers, injecting fat that is harvested from the abdomen or flanks into the lower eyelid area. Typically, in these procedures, 70 percent of the fat will be incorporated, producing a long-lasting outcome (for more details on fat transfers, see Chapter 5).

Avoid injecting non-hyaluronic acid fillers since they can often result in visible lumps, nodules, and irregularities. On the other hand, as you now know, hyaluronic acid can be reversed if the results aren't satisfactory (see Chapter 5).

Surgical Eyelid Lifts (Blepharoplasty)

For All Ethnicities

There are a few different approaches a surgeon may take when it comes to upper and lower eyelid surgery. In traditional upper blepharoplasty, a hidden incision is placed within the natural creases of the eyelid, called the supratarsal crease, making it virtually invisible once fully healed (Figure 22). Through this incision, excess skin, muscle, and fat are removed.

For the lower eyelids, the procedure requires one of a few different approaches, depending on how the skin and fat are aging around the lower eyelids. A lower blepharoplasty is done

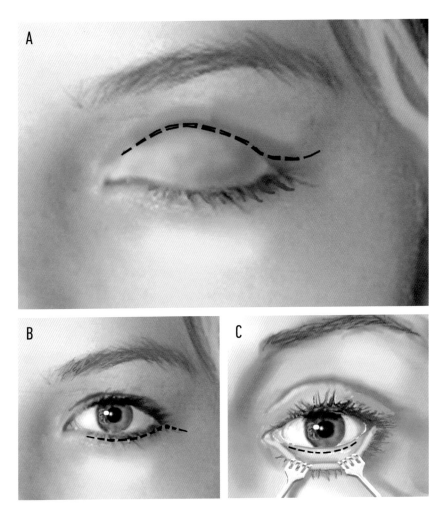

Figure 22: Location of eyelid lift incision. A) The incision for an upper eyelid lift is hidden in the upper eyelid crease and a "crow's foot wrinkle." B) Lower eyelid lift to remove excess skin is placed 2 mm below the eyelashes. C) Lower eyelid incision from inside the eyelid called a "transconjunctival" incision when fat bags under the eyes need work but no skin removal is necessary.

Natural-Appearing Versus Overdone Eyelid Lifts

When done with a heavy hand, upper eyelid lifts performed in the West Coast style can create an over-exaggerated open eye by removing all the upper eyelid fat and dramatically reducing the skin and muscle. The approach is characterized by its resulting deep upper eyelid crease, which looks carved out rather than soft. For patients who prefer a more natural result, I have modified the traditional upper eyelid surgery to a more subtle East Coast aesthetic. I call it the "conservation upper eyelid lift."

To perform a conservation upper eyelid lift, I ask all of my patients to bring me photos of themselves at a younger age so that I restore only what they once had instead of creating something that never existed before. To avoid removing excessive amounts of skin, I mark the patient while he or she is sitting upright with eyes closed, which allows me to calculate how much extra skin to remove while still permitting the upper eyelids to close naturally. Once the incisions are made, I do not remove any muscle from the eyelid crease, so that a natural amount of fullness persists.

When we look at an iconic young Hollywood actress, such as Jennifer Lawrence, we can see that there is a natural fullness under her eyebrows—a signature of youth that we want to maintain. There are two fat pads that can be modified in the upper eyelid: the central fat pad, above the center of the eyelid, and the nasal fat pad, close to the inner corner of the eye. The West Coast–style procedure completely removes these two fat pads, creating an overly sculpted look. To create natural

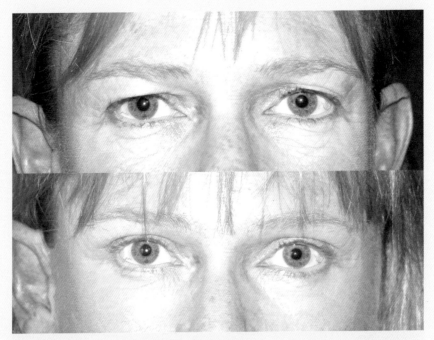

Figure 23: Before (top) and after (bottom) of a woman who had a conservation upper eyelid lift, preserving the natural fat of the upper eyelid and resulting in a softer and more natural result. This method avoids overly open, sculpted-appearing eyelids.

contours, the central fat pad should be only slightly reduced. Preserving more of this fat creates soft contours that appear unmanipulated. Finally, tiny stiches close up the incisions and are removed within the next few days (Figure 23).

Similarly, for lower eyelids, the West Coast style removes fat bags from under the eyes, causing a carved-out look that accentuates the tear trough. The East Coast style maintains volume by simply moving the fat pads from where we don't want them to the tear trough, so that the dark circles are filled. These fat pads have their blood supply intact, and are stitched into position so they cannot move, meaning they will last a lifetime. This fat transposition (different from the fat transfers/stem cell procedures that inject body fat harvested from other areas of the body, which makes it impossible to predict how much fat will be naturally reabsorbed) can be performed through an external or internal incision. Filling in the tear troughs creates a smooth transition from the eyelid to the cheek, which is the hallmark of youth. The friends of my patients rave about how great they look but are unable to pinpoint exactly why (Figure 24). I have published this technique in *JAMA Facial Plastic Surgery* to help popularize this approach with facial plastic surgeons.[1]

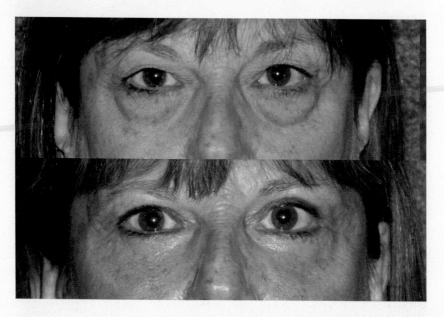

Figure 24: Before (top) and after (bottom) of a woman who had a lower eyelid lift with transposition (moving) of the fat bags into the lower eyelid hollows (dark circles), creating a smooth, youthful contour starting at the lower eyelid and blending to the upper cheek.

with either an external incision in the skin or with an internal incision inside the eyelid (Figure 22C). The external incision technique is used when extra skin needs to be removed, in which case the incision is placed 1 millimeter away from the lower eyelash line. This provides access to any excessive muscle and fat, allowing for the skin to be trimmed and tightened. Extremely fine sutures are then used to meticulously close the incisions, which minimizes any visible scarring. If you just have mild to moderate skin excess, the skin can be tightened with a fractional CO_2 laser (see Chapter 4), often referred to as a laser eyelid lift.

The internal, or transconjunctival, blepharoplasty technique is performed when there is no need for excess skin removal, in which case an incision is made inside the eyelid through the lining of the eye to access the excess muscle and fat. This transconjunctival technique is often used on younger patients who have not yet developed excess skin.

Upper and lower eyelid surgery usually lasts approximately twenty years, so there is no maintenance required. For most, it is a once-in-a-lifetime procedure, though it can be touched up years later, if desired.

UNIQUE CHARACTERISTICS FOR ASIAN EYES

Asian blepharoplasty, or double-eyelid surgery, is the procedure that places a crease in Asian eyes that genetically don't possess one. Before surgery, the eyelid skin naturally folds over the upper eyelids, making the eyelid aperture appear narrower. This fold is called an epicanthal fold.   The anatomical reason for this is the skin lacks a ligament that attaches the eyelid skin to the cartilage under the eyelid crease. This surgery is very common in some Asian countries, particularly in Korea. The operation has a similar incision to that used in traditional upper eyelid lifts, but the skin is sutured to the cartilage so that a crease is formed.

I've found that very few of my middle-aged Asian patients want to change the overall character of their eyelids that the double eyelid surgery creates. Rather, they've noticed that their eyelid skin has begun to droop, and they want to restore their prior appearance. I am much less aggressive with skin removal in these cases and do not create any connection of the skin to the eyelid crease (Figure 25).

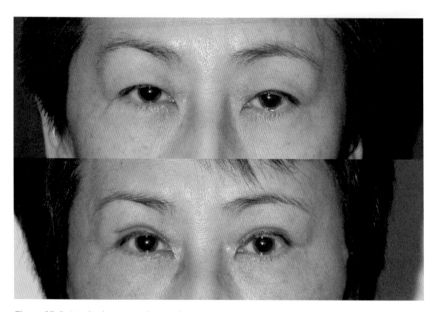

Figure 25: Before (top) and after (bottom) of a female Asian patient who had an upper eyelid lift. The natural fold of the eye, called an epicanthal fold, should be preserved in these cases to maintain the patient's facial ethnic identity.

EYELID SURGERY FOR MEN

Many men seek eyelid rejuvenation to continue to project a youthful and energetic appearance in the workplace. Especially in the business world, people associate an older appearance with a diminishing ability.

The male and female eyelid anatomies are different, including the shape of the eyes, meaning the approach to eyelid surgery for male patients is different from that of their female counterparts. In male upper eyelid surgery, I preserve a natural masculine eyelid by not removing all the redundant skin, instead leaving a little excess, like that you would see in a thirty-year-old male. It is also important not to overly resect or deepen the upper eyelid crease. This is accomplished by removing fat only from the upper eyelid nasal fat pad, closer to the nose, and not from the central fat pad of the upper eyelids (which is routinely performed in female upper eyelid lifts).

In male lower eyelid surgery, there are broad, tight ligaments around the tear trough called the orbitomalar ligaments, which must be released before the excess skin is removed. If they are not released, the lower eyelids will appear tight, which looks altered and feminized. Similar to female blepharoplasty, the fat bags are then repositioned into the dark circles under the eyes to help keep the eyes from looking hollow and to give a more youthful appearance (Figure 26).

Singer Kenny Rogers is one of the most notorious victims of a botched male eyelid lift (combined with a forehead/brow lift). It altered the shape of his eyes and completely changed his appearance. What went wrong? The fat in his upper eyelids

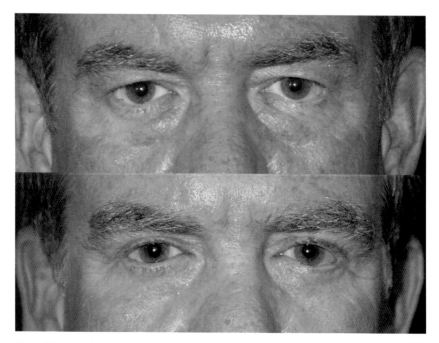

Figure 26: Before (top) and after (bottom) of a male patient with upper and lower eyelid lifts. Notice how he looks refreshed yet masculine even though the brows are slightly heavy. Less skin and fat are removed to maintain masculinity. Brow lifts often create a feminized appearance and should be avoided—a heavier brow is attractive in men.

was completely *excavated*. Carving out all of the fat leaves the eyelids looking feminine and rounded. In addition, Rogers seems to have experienced the most common problem in lower blepharoplasty—what's called *ectropion*, where the lower eyelid gets pulled down and the shape of the eye becomes unnaturally rounded (see lower eyelid lift complications on page 146). Rogers has lovely, big eyes now, which would look wonderful on a woman but perhaps not ideal on a man, especially one whose entrenched notions of masculinity inform his identity.

BOTCHED UPPER EYELID SURGERY: WHAT CAN GO WRONG AND HOW TO FIX IT

If a doctor isn't careful to take a conservative approach with upper eyelid surgery (instead believing "more is more"), he or she might take away too much skin, leaving their patients unable to fully close their eyes. This condition is called lagophthalmos and leads to severely dry and irritated eyes. The only way to fix this problem is with a more complex reconstructive surgery in which we harvest skin grafts, usually from the skin behind the ear, and place them back into the upper eyelids. Thankfully repair is possible, but the recovery is long, taking four to six weeks until the initial healing is complete (Figure 27).

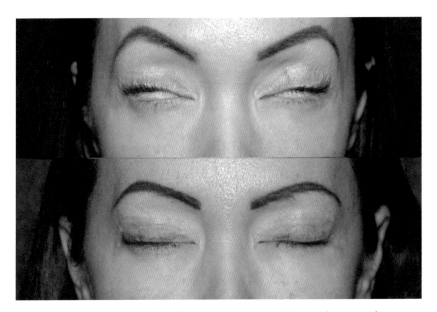

Figure 27: Before (top) and after (bottom) of a female patient who had corrective surgery for excess skin removal from an upper eyelid lift (performed elsewhere), causing her not to be able to close her eyes—a condition called lagophthalmos. This mistake was corrected by replacing upper eyelid skin with skin grafts borrowed from behind the ears.

Another problem that can occur is something I call "curtain call." Many surgeons will not pass the outer corner of the eye when they are excising skin so that after surgery the hooding under the eyebrow remains. If the incision stops short at the outer corner of the eye, the extra hooded skin that is left behind can get bunched up like the curtain-call drapery pulled across the stage at the end of a Broadway show. The incision should go past the outer corner of the eye and continue into a natural wrinkle of the patient's crow's feet so that all the hooded skin under the eyebrow can be removed. Plastic surgical suturing makes this incision almost invisible.

When too much upper eyelid fat is removed, a deep sulcus, or furrow, is created above the eyelid crease that can look harsh. This soft tissue padding can be re-created using fat grafting to replace it. What's great about fat grafting is that it is performed by injecting fat through a cannula that is approximately the width of a needle, so it requires no incision. Remember, what makes people look youthful is their soft tissue padding around the upper eyelids (Figure 28).

BOTCHED LOWER EYELID SURGERY: WHAT CAN GO WRONG AND HOW TO FIX IT

For most lower eyelid surgery cases, it is important *not* to remove the fat bags under the eyes but rather to transpose or move the fat into the deep grooving and hollows that appear as dark circles. Most surgeons still remove these fat bags, creating deep-set eyes that are a telltale sign of surgery. *Removing* fat causes the perceived length of the lower eyelid to increase and

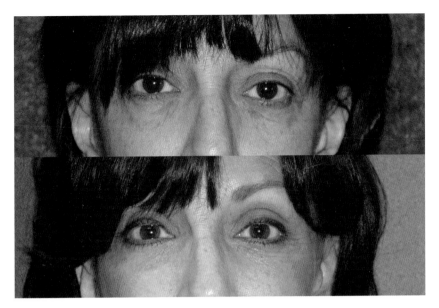

Figure 28: Before (top) and after (bottom) of a female patient who had corrective surgery for excess fat removal from an upper and lower eyelid lift (performed elsewhere) that created a sunken-looking eye. This was corrected by injecting fat borrowed from the abdomen into the upper and lower eyelids.

look older, just in a different way. Because of this tendency, I have performed hundreds of cases of fat transfers to the lower eyelids after patients have had the volume removed from their lower eyelids. Because they have already had their lower eyelid skin removed and tightened, this can also be accomplished by injecting cannulas (in which case no incision or stitching is required).

Another technique to be wary of is canthoplasty, a procedure that is common in the West Coast style. Many surgeons perform this procedure with a lower eyelid lift. The canthus, or outer corner of the eyelid, is stitched up on a slant, creating a "cat eye." If patients want this look, great. If not, it can be upsetting. It's a problem that is difficult to correct, requiring reopening the eyelid incision and relaxing the corner of the eye by releasing the sutures placed to hold it in that position. My advice is to have a discussion with your surgeon before eyelid surgery expressing your desire to avoid the cat-eye outcome. If you *do* want this look, make sure you ask your doctor so that it is incorporated into your procedure.

When doctors don't tighten the lower eyelid muscles to support the lower eyelid, or when they remove too much skin, the lower eyelid pulls down, creating an ectropion—that "hound dog" look. Ectropion can be repaired, but all of the available revision procedures can be complex. They include repeating the lower eyelid incision and tightening the lower eyelid

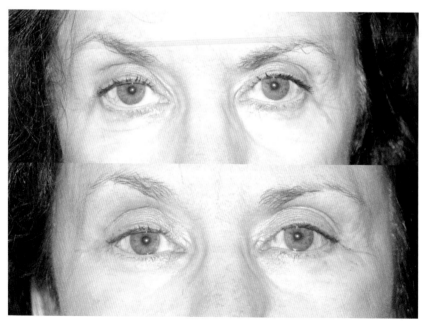

Figure 29: Before (top) and after (bottom) of a female patient who had corrective surgery for excess skin removal during an eyelid lift (performed elsewhere) that created pulled down, "hound dog"–looking eyes, a condition called ectropion. I corrected it by performing a revision lower eyelid lift and tightening the lower eyelid with a procedure called a canthoplasty.

Eyelid Lift Versus Brow Lift: Self-Diagnosing the Problem

Sometimes the upper eyelids appear droopy, but the problem is not, in fact, your eyelids but your forehead and brow. When the forehead drops, the eyebrows fall on top of the upper eyelids like a window shade. The best way to decide for yourself if the problem lies with your eyelids or your forehead is to sit in front of the mirror and lift the forehead with your fingers, just above the eyebrows. If you like what you see, you do not need an upper eyelid lift but a brow lift. For some, both an upper eyelid lift and a brow lift should be done at the same time for maximum results, but this can best be determined by a plastic surgeon you trust.

tendons, skin grafting to replace the excessive skin removal, or endoscopic midface surgery, which can help support the lower eyelids by lifting the cheeks (Figure 29).

What Happens to Your Forehead/Brow as You Age

As you get older, thanks to sun exposure and the inevitable pull of gravity, the skin on your forehead begins to sag, resulting in frown lines, wrinkles, and increased heaviness of the eyebrows and upper eyelids. These changes can make you look tired, angry, or sad, even when you're full of energy, calm, and happy.

Nonsurgical Forehead/Brow Procedures

BOTOX

Botox is one of the easiest and least-invasive procedures readily available to treat wrinkles and drooping in your forehead. (Of course, sometimes I think it's almost *too* available, as any licensed physician or even dentist can offer Botox to their patients, which doesn't mean they're well trained or that they *should*.) With just a few injections, your lines and wrinkles will literally disappear—temporarily, at least. That's because, as you learned in Chapter 5, Botox works by blocking the impulses from your nerves to your tiny facial muscles that are related to your expression lines. After the injections, your underlying muscles relax and your overlying skin remains smooth and unwrinkled.

The great thing about Botox is that when it's done with a judicial and skilled hand, you won't look totally frozen or unnaturally smooth. Untreated muscles are still able to contract, so you should still be able to smile, laugh, frown, or squint naturally. The only drawback is that Botox only lasts for three to five months. For a more permanent improvement, especially on the frown lines between the eyebrows, you might be better off in the long run with an endoscopic brow lift.

Surgical Forehead/Brow Lifts

For All Ethnicities

I've found that many of my patients are very apprehensive about forehead/brow procedures because they've seen so many botched results that leave people looking unnaturally startled or surprised. This is a common result when proportions get out of whack. Eyebrows naturally follow a curve, so when they're off-kilter, it is particularly noticeable and off-putting. With more traditional brow lifting techniques, both ends of the eyebrow (both closer to the nose and closer to the ear) end up being at the same height, making the eyes appear unnaturally wide open, staring, or even surprised. The best way to make sure that you and your surgeon share the same aesthetic is to suggest reviewing your desired brow position in the mirror together. Hold your brows in position with your fingers and actually have the doctor measure the amount of elevation you desire at the inner, center, and outer corners of the brow with a caliper (a plastic surgery measuring device) or a millimeter ruler.

There are two techniques for forehead/brow surgery: traditional and endoscopic (Figure 30). With either of these techniques, a brow lift can last for ten to fifteen years. With a traditional brow lift, a long incision is made, running across the top of the head from one ear to the other. Not surprisingly, the traditional lift leaves a long scar and has a much longer recovery than an endoscopic procedure. Side effects include numbness of the scalp that feels like there is a permanent cap on the top of the head.

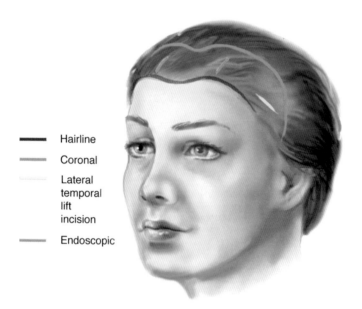

Hairline

Coronal

Lateral
temporal
lift
incision

Endoscopic

Figure 30: Illustration demonstrating the incisions used in different types of brow lift surgery. The main types include coronal, hairline, endoscopic, and lateral temporal brow lifts.

Generally speaking, an endoscopic or keyhole brow lift is a better and less painful option. Endoscopic simply means "telescopic." Through a few small incisions in the hairline just large enough to pass the endoscope (which is the width of a drinking straw), the surgeon is able to reposition your forehead with more precision as he or she lifts the drooping brows, flattens any forehead wrinkles, and makes the eyes seem bigger. The muscles that cause the frown lines and the "elevens" between the eyebrows can also be removed, which can help prevent the need for repeat Botox injections. During this surgery, I re-create natural proportions, lifting the center of the brow only slightly but lifting higher at the outer aspect, which creates a feminine arch that my patients love (Figure 31). If

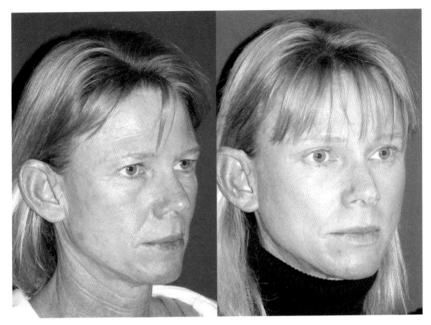

Figure 31: Before (left) and after (right) of a woman who had an endoscopic brow lift. Notice how the outer third of the brow is more elevated, creating a natural look. This avoids the startled appearance of old-style brow lifts. She also had an upper and lower eyelid lift performed at the same time.

the center of the brow does not need to be elevated, I perform a lateral temporal lift, which only lifts the outer corner of the eyebrow. This procedure is more common in younger patients in their forties and early fifties who do not need as much.

If your hairline is positioned farther back than normal (otherwise known as a high forehead), an endoscopic brow lift may not be the best procedure for you. The endoscopic procedure will elevate the hairline further in those with long foreheads and high hairlines. Instead, the better approach utilizes an incision made just in front of the hairline (termed a pre-trichial brow lift). During this procedure, both the forehead and brows can be lifted and the hairline lowered so that the forehead is shortened. Lowering the hairline always makes you look more youthful. The incisions are designed to make the final scar barely visible.

FOREHEAD/BROW LIFTS FOR MEN

I have a firm position about brow lifts for men: Don't do them! When we look at the brow position of iconic Hollywood stars, such as Brad Pitt or Tom Cruise, we see their brows are heavy. It's a good thing, as men with high testosterone levels have what's called frontal bossing, where the area over their brow appears more significant. A heavier brow accentuates the bridge of bone in the forehead right above the eyes properly known as the supraorbital ridge, a male facial skeletal characteristic. Because this ridge becomes accentuated with age, it's one of the reasons that men are often said to become more handsome and distinguished as they get older. The eyebrow orientation in men should go straight across this part of the forehead, as it also accentuates the bony ridge. Too much of an arch above the bone is a stereotypical female orientation. The only man I know who gets away with this is Jack Nicholson, who has unique, naturally arched brows, but you have to admit he does have a permanently quizzical look that, fortunately for him, suits his personality.

This is what I explain to men who ask for a brow lift. I'll recommend it only if their brows have fallen low enough that they start to affect and obstruct vision. Usually, upper eyelid surgery is a much better choice if their lids are heavy or drooping, leaving them looking tired or angry all the time.

BOTCHED FOREHEAD/BROW LIFTS: WHAT CAN GO WRONG AND HOW TO FIX IT

If a plastic surgeon is too aggressive and over-elevates the brow and forehead during brow lift surgery, the result can look artificial, leaving you with a too-smooth forehead and a perpetually surprised expression. Even an endoscopic brow lift can create this look if the surgeon is overzealous.

A botched brow lift can be fixed in what's called a brow-lift reversal, but it is a very significant operation (surgeon code for a long, difficult, and painful procedure). Your surgeon will have to make an incision, lift the scalp back, drill holes in the skull, and then move the hair-bearing portion of your scalp a

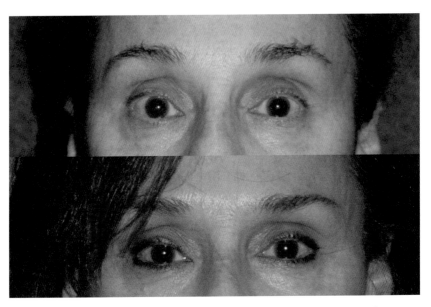

Figure 32: Before (top) and after (bottom) of a female patient who had corrective surgery for an overdone brow lift (performed elsewhere) that makes the eyes look surprised and too widely open. The brow lift reversal procedure involves moving the scalp and forehead back down and securing to the forehead bone.

little bit forward. This allows the forehead and brow to move back down, taking some of the lift off the brows and placing them in a more natural position or even back to where they started. Fortunately, the incision is typically made along the front of the hairline, which tends to heal very nicely, with little visible scarring, if done carefully with specialized plastic surgery suturing techniques (Figure 32).

What to Expect After Eyelid and Forehead/Brow Surgery

These procedures are done on an outpatient basis, with local anesthesia or twilight anesthesia. Twilight anesthesia is the same anesthesia that you get during a colonoscopy. We never use general anesthesia, so patients do not wake up nauseated (see Chapter 12 for more on anesthesia).

Immediately following surgery, patients should expect some slight swelling, bruising, and redness around the incision sites, which goes away after a few days. Be aware that lower eyelid surgery causes much more bruising than upper eyelid surgery—you can get big shiners around your eyes that take longer to fade. Bruising after upper eyelid surgery usually fades after four to five days; bruising after lower eyelid surgery fades after seven to ten days. Whether you had an upper or lower eyelid procedure, your eyelids will generally feel tight, with some soreness, which can be treated with a prescription pain reliever. Common side effects can include tearing, dry eye, and sensitivity to light that is treated with a lubricating ointment.

Avoid activities that can dry the eyes, such as wearing contacts and extended computer or tablet use. Wear dark sunglasses whenever you go outside to avoid any irritations that may be caused by the sun and wind. To help reduce the swelling, gently place a cold compress over your eyes. Use lubricating eye drops to keep your eyes from drying out. During the first week of recovery, it is important to keep your head elevated as much as possible, which will help minimize bruising and swelling. Avoid any strenuous activities that increase blood flow to the head or eyes, including bending, hanging upside down, heavy lifting, sports, and any kind of cardio workouts, for at least two to three weeks after your procedure.

An endoscopic brow lift offers the advantage of a quick recovery—usually no more than five to seven days. All incisions are hidden behind the hairline, so that they are not visible to anyone, and there is less bruising, swelling, and lingering numbness. A traditional brow lift, on the other hand, will usually take seven to ten days to resolve bruising. A temporal headache is common for the first twenty-four to forty-eight hours and can be treated with Tylenol. You cannot use ibuprofen because it will increase your likelihood of bleeding.

Like all the procedures discussed in this book, eyelid and forehead/brow lifts are only as good as the surgeon who performs them. But when you've done your research and found a qualified doctor who understands your needs, there is no need to fear them. Read on for other safe, effective procedures that address the nose, chin, lips, and neck—all of which this section will cover in detail.

1 Andrew A. Jacono and Melanie H. Malone, "Extended Submuscular Blepharoplasty with Orbitomalar Ligament Release and Orbital Fat Repositioning," *JAMA Facial Plastic Surgery* 19, no. 1 (2017), 72–73, doi: 10.1001/jamafacial.2016.1047, https://www.ncbi.nlm.nih.gov/pubmed/27606774.

7 Perfect Your Nose

If your eyes are the first feature that people notice when they meet you, your nose is the second. But while plastic surgery on your eyes is considered risky due to its potential to change what is familiar about your face, plastic surgery on your nose is often intended to do just that—it changes the character of your face in a positive way, bringing about balance. Even a slight alteration can greatly improve your appearance; when you look at before-and-after photographs of good nose jobs, or rhinoplasties, the results can be astonishing. People look younger, more balanced, more beautiful. It can seem that every other feature on their face has also been changed—when, of course, all that shifted was the facial proportions you read about in Chapter 2. It can make the face look slimmer, the cheekbones higher, the eyes more open and beautiful.

How will you know if a nose job is right for you? Take your time before you decide. Noses are incredibly diverse, and sometimes having a distinctive nose gives a face a unique character. This is what the actress Jennifer Grey, who made an indelible impression in the 1987 hit film *Dirty Dancing* (not just for her acting opposite the late Patrick Swayze but for her unique nose), discovered, to her regret, when she decided to have surgery. "I went into the operating room a celebrity and came out anonymous," she famously admitted. "I'll always be this once-famous actress nobody recognizes because of a nose job."[1]

And yet, rhinoplasty can be done in such a stealthy fashion that my nose job patients often tell me that after surgery everyone they know remarks on how great they look, asking if they've changed their hair style or color, or lost weight, but never suspecting a change to their nose. Their own closest friends and even family members can't get over how great they look but cannot ascribe it to rhinoplasty.

My patients' requests vary dramatically, but it's important to discuss with them how they can get the nose they really want that also matches their face and proportions. If someone has a broad face and you create an itty-bitty nose, it can actually make the face look even larger. Some patients want sculptural noses or aquiline noses, which might be perfect for some face shapes, but on others might draw too much attention away from their other features. Sometimes they want a nose like a particular celebrity; sometimes they have ethnic considerations and want a nose that looks typically representative of their own culture. And some patients just want a small bump removed, with no other changes.

Today, patients have the amazing option of having their nose altered with either a nonsurgical or a surgical approach. Bridges can be straightened, tips lifted and refined, all without surgery! Injecting hyaluronic acid filler to reshape the nose is often referred to as a nonsurgical rhinoplasty and is discussed in more detail below. The disadvantage to this procedure is its temporary nature, and there are limitations to how much change the doctor can nonsurgically effect.

The last thing you want is to have your procedure done by a surgeon whose cookie-cutter approach leaves every single one of his patients with the exact same nose. You'll notice this right away when you take the time to assess the doctor's before-and-after photos. This is one of the reasons I use digital photography and computer imaging software to simulate how patients will look after surgery. It's extremely helpful for patients to see exactly how their new nose will look, and for us to discuss all the details prior to their surgery.

Understanding Your Nasal Anatomy Before Rhinoplasty

The nose is made of paired nasal bones and cartilages on the left and right sides of the nose. The nose can be broken down into an upper, middle, and lower third, with the upper third of the nose made up of the nasal bones, the middle third of the nose made up of upper lateral cartilages, and the lower third made up of lower lateral cartilages (Figure 33).

The nasal bridge is made up of contributions from the nasal bones and upper lateral cartilages and the nasal tip is made

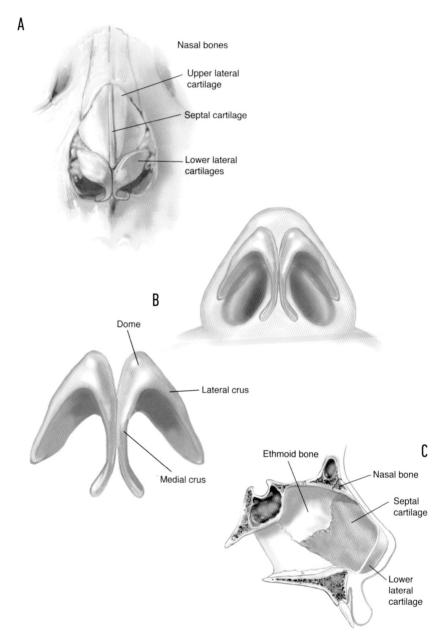

Figure 33: The anatomy of the nose. A) The nasal bones and upper lateral cartilages create the bridge. B) The lower lateral cartilages create the tip, with the dome section defining the tip of the nose. C) The nasal septum is inside the nose and made of cartilage that can be used to add to the nose during rhinoplasty.

A Picture Is Worth a Thousand Words: Digital Morphing

No matter how carefully and thoroughly I describe my approach to a rhinoplasty, I'll have more success communicating and my patient will be able to show me what he or she wants if I create the nose digitally with computer imaging, using his or her own face. The digital image also gives me the ability to really fine-tune the aesthetic according to what the patient desires, including specific changes to the tip of the nose or the curve of the bridge. It's like trying on a dress before you buy it.

I also encourage patients to bring pictures of a few noses they like that I can work from; most commonly, patients choose photos of a family member, an Instagram model, or a celebrity. Many of my colleagues don't engage in this practice, discouraging patients from bringing photos featuring noses they like, because they feel it creates an unrealistic expectation. I do not promise my patients the exact nose they desire because so often it would not fit their face, but if I see that they like a shorter nose that is ever so slightly upturned, it helps me incorporate that detail into their morphing. In the end, the patient decides what he or she wants, but my guidance, with the help of digital morphing, steers them out of trouble.

up of the lower lateral cartilages. Too much of either of these components makes a bump on the bridge. The lower lateral cartilages have three main defined areas: the lateral crus, which makes up the side of the nasal tip; the dome area, which is the tip-defining point; and the medial crus, which makes up the center of the nose under the tip (called the columella). Too much cartilage in any of these areas will create a wide, droopy, or poorly defined tip.

Internal to the nose is the nasal septum, which is a thin piece of cartilage (the thickness of a credit card) that separates the left and right side of the nose internally. The lower lateral cartilages connect to the septum, and too much septal cartilage will make the nose look long. Interestingly, cartilage can be borrowed from the septum, removed to be used in surgical rhinoplasty to build up or support the nose in different areas, but this does not affect the function of the nose. In fact, when people get their "deviated septum" fixed, twisted cartilage is removed to make the nose breathe better.

What Happens to Your Nose as You Age

As we age, unavoidable changes occur to our noses. I do a lot of rhinoplasties on patients as they approach forty and older. They show me photographs of their noses from their twenties and early thirties, which look completely different from their noses on the day they arrive in my office. This is perfectly normal—even if other features remain youthful, the nose can't help but show signs of aging, mainly because of gravity.

Inevitably, with time, your nose becomes longer and the tip droops. When this happens, it will accentuate any bumps in the bridge. Additionally, the ligaments that keep the left and right nasal tip cartilages together loosen and the tip cartilages become wider, making the nasal tip look wider and bulbous. As the tip widens, the nostrils flare more. All of these changes make the whole face look longer, broader, and wider, bringing more attention to the lower third of the face. The unfortunate result is that it will draw more attention to drooping, including the nasolabial folds and early jowls that can make the face look older.

Nonsurgical Nose Job (Liquid Rhinoplasty)

A nonsurgical nose job (or nonsurgical rhinoplasty) is a very common procedure that is done using injectable hyaluronic acid fillers and Botox. Controlled, precise injections can make the nose look more proportional and even lift up a drooping tip. The results are instantaneous with essentially no recovery time, unlike with surgery. I have had patients nonsurgically alter their nose a few days before an important event, date, or photoshoot. On average, the results last about one year. Although this option is a welcome alternative to surgery, it does have limitations, so you should make sure that you understand what the procedure can and can't accomplish, and adjust your expectations accordingly (Figure 34).

Botox can lift up a droopy tip, which can be caused by an overactive depressor septi muscle that pulls down the nasal

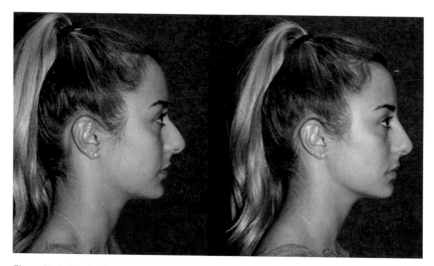

Figure 34: Before (left) and after (right) of a female patient who had a nonsurgical "liquid rhino-plasty" to reduce the hump in the nasal bridge, straightening it, and to lift and redefine her nasal tip.

tip, especially when smiling. When injected in between the nostrils on the undersurface of the nose, this muscle releases, creating a more upturned nose. Botox works right away and lasts from three to five months. Fillers can also be added where the nose meets the lip to support the tip at its base. Using both of these techniques together gives the best results, but the reality is that it lifts the tip by only 2 to 3 millimeters at best, which is not very much. I recommend doing this only if your tip requires a small amount of lifting. Anyone with a heavy or droopier tip will usually not see a significant enough difference to make it worth the expense, in which case surgery is a better option.

There are many ways we can reshape the nose with hyaluronic acid injectable fillers. I almost always use Restylane for noses, since it can be easily reversed with one treatment of an injectable enzyme called hyaluronidase. It is rare, but sometimes patients want to reduce the amount of work done or even remove it completely. Other hyaluronic acid fillers may take several sessions of enzyme injections to be reversed.

The most common use for filler in a nonsurgical rhinoplasty is to diminish a hump or bump on the bridge of the nose. Filler placed into the bridge above the area of the bump makes it appear straighter. Bear in mind, however, that this cannot make the bridge smaller or create a more feminine curve in the bridge. Only surgery can do that. If the bridge is crooked to one side, you can fill the opposite side of the nasal bridge it bends away from to camouflage the twisting. If you have a flat bridge, fillers can augment it. This is a very common request from Asian and African American patients who often have flatter noses. Unlike with nasal bumps, this treatment can give results that are more similar to rhinoplasty surgery, which uses either your own cartilage or a permanent implant to build up the bridge, instead of a temporary injection. The only difference is that fillers are temporary and surgery is permanent. Having filler is a good choice for patients who want to see and live with the results before opting for a permanent fix.

Injecting filler into the nose is like sculpting, and, depending on who is doing it, the results can be under- or overdone, or they can appear lumpy or asymmetric. These problems can be corrected using additional filler injections, or by dissolving some away. A dreaded but extremely rare complication occurs when the blood supply to the nasal skin is compromised with the injections, causing the nasal skin to scar. After injections, if your nasal skin turns white, gray, or dark purple (not like a bruise), your nasal blood supply may have been affected. Take an aspirin (325 milligrams) to increase blood flow and contact your doctor immediately to dissolve away product to prevent permanent scarring.

Surgical Nose Job (Rhinoplasty)
For All Ethnicities

Rhinoplasty can completely reshape and refine a nose, from the bridge to the tip. You can adjust any part of it or all of it, depending on its shape and how it fits your face—from a very small and nearly imperceptible reduction of a little bump or slightly drooping tip, to a complete alteration, making a disproportionately large, hooked, flat, or wide nose smaller, slimmer, smoother, and more elegant.

There are two main approaches in nose reshaping surgery: open and closed rhinoplasty. Open rhinoplasty involves a

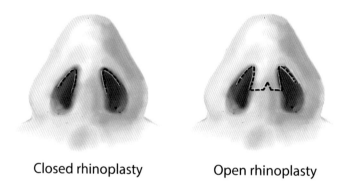

Closed rhinoplasty   Open rhinoplasty

Figure 35: Illustration of the incisions for a closed versus open rhinoplasty. The closed approach has internal incisions inside the nostrils and no external incisions. The open approach has a small incision that connects the two nostril incisions of the closed rhinoplasty to give more exposure to the nasal tip, allowing for more nasal "tip work."

small incision across the base of the nose, after which the skin of the nasal tip is flipped up like the hood of a car. A closed or endo-nasal rhinoplasty involves making the incisions inside the nose, so there won't be a visible scar (Figure 35).

Most primary or first-time rhinoplasties can be accomplished using either approach, depending on the doctor's background and training. Most surgeons in the United States only perform open rhinoplasty surgeries, as this is what they're trained to do—it allows them to easily see the nasal contours and cartilage during the procedure. I do both open and closed and choose the best approach depending on the goals of the surgery. Some modifications of the nose, especially certain nasal tip maneuvers, can only be done with an open rhinoplasty approach. Open rhinoplasty is best when a patient has a large nose that sticks out or projects from their face (called an over-projected nose), when a lot of cartilage grafting is needed (it's harder to put the grafts in with closed rhinoplasty), when a nasal tip needs to be built up and supported, or when a previous surgery is being revised.

Each approach has its advantages and disadvantages. There are several drawbacks to open rhinoplasty: It takes longer to perform (up to and over an hour longer) than a closed rhinoplasty; there may also be some additional scarring and thickening of the nasal tip that results from the more extensive surgical dissection of the nasal skin; and swelling and recovery require a longer healing time. With closed rhinoplasty, there is significantly less post-operative swelling, better nasal tip support, a shorter operating time needing less anesthesia, and speedier recovery. The disadvantage to the closed approach is that there are some limitations to how much nasal tip refinement you can accomplish. For patients who require nasal cartilage tip grafting or need more nasal tip support, the open approach is the way to go.

With either approach, experienced rhinoplasty surgeons are able to reshape the nose. For the bridge, the excess nasal bone and upper lateral cartilage are removed to smooth the profile. Sculpting the nasal bones of the bridge by shaving rather than breaking the nose is a technique that will dramatically decrease post-surgical recovery time. (Breaking the bones is what causes bruises around the eyes, which can take a few weeks to resolve.) For the tip, the lower lateral cartilages are shaped using sutures that help refine and narrow the dome region. This technique is better to use than cutting away the lower lateral cartilage, which is the tip supportive structure—cutting too much of the cartilage will destabilize the nose and make it more likely to collapse and cause problems.

While some people idolize nasal tips that are small, piggy, and pinched, which comes from removing the lower lateral cartilages, my Park Avenue patients specifically tell me they do not want this exaggerated result. The suturing and reshaping of the tip cartilages described refines and reshapes the cartilages without making them too small. Some patients with extremely droopy tip cartilages that are weak and floppy will require a nasal tip graft, which lifts, supports, and defines the tip (Figure 36).

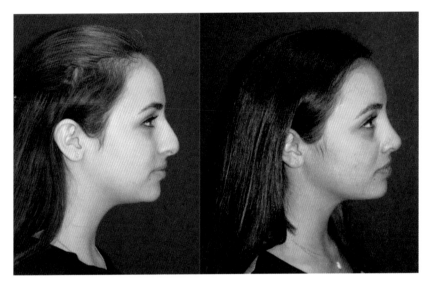

Figure 36: Before (left) and after (right) of a female patient who had a closed rhinoplasty to lift and define the nasal tip. She had her bridge reduced, creating a gentle curve at the same time.

Ultrasonic Rhinoplasty

The most advanced, state-of-the-art way to reduce the bridge is with ultrasonic rhinoplasty. Instead of using a chisel or rasp (file) to mechanically reduce humps or bumps, this machine uses a crystal that vibrates at an ultra-high frequency. There are currently two devices on the market—the Piezo and the Sonopet. The equipment will very gently sculpt bone and cartilage, but as soon as it touches soft tissues, it ceases to cut and instead just vibrates in place. You can reduce the bridge more precisely with this device, resulting in less trauma and thus less bruising.

The nasal bridge is one place where I see big differences between West Coast and East Coast aesthetics. The ski slope is popular amongst young starlets in Hollywood who want to look like they've had their noses done. If you prefer a more subtle approach, I can create a slight but gentle curve more precisely with the ultrasonic device that would leave people raving about your appearance but without knowing you had surgery. With an ultrasonic rhinoplasty, there is no need to break the bones to reduce the nasal bridge width (Figure 37). Most surgeons who have not invested in this technology use a hammer.

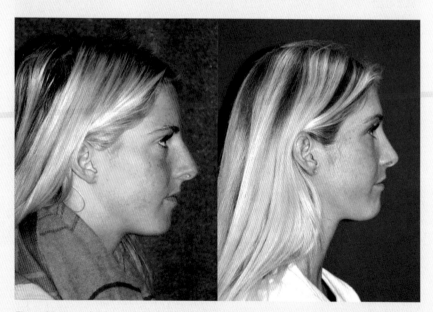

Figure 37: Before (left) and after (right) of a female patient who had an ultrasonic rhinoplasty to reduce a hump of the nasal bridge. This minimally invasive technique uses a small incision inside the nose and an ultrasonic tool to precisely reduce the nasal bridge.

The Teenage Nose

I spend a lot of time talking to my potential rhinoplasty patients, as they tend to be younger than patients who come in for other procedures such as facelifts or eyelid surgery. Many of them are teenagers, and they're at the age when a crooked, bumpy, unusually shaped, or overly large nose can make a serious dent in self-confidence. Rhinoplasty can be a physically and emotionally satisfying operation for teenagers when their motivations and expectations are realistic. When I tell them that a good rhinoplasty can free them from having to think about their nose every time they take a selfie, their relief is palpable. They're even happier when they see the results.

Rhinoplasties are, in fact, the number-one surgical procedure requested by teenagers. But, if your teenager is thinking about this procedure, make sure you discuss the real reasons behind their decision. Your teen should be self-motivated to improve their appearance solely to feel better about themselves—not because they want to please their parents, fit in with their peers, or look more like a specific celebrity.

A nose job will *not* be the panacea to the angst of teenage life. It will, however, improve the nose aesthetically, creating better harmony with other facial features, which often helps with self-esteem. I've seen so many of my teenaged patients blossom and work harder in school, become more socially connected with their peers, and seemingly grow up overnight because their new appearance gives them the confidence to excel. It can actually change their lives in so many ways for the better, but it is a big decision that should not be taken lightly.

UNIQUE CHARACTERISTICS FOR RHINOPLASTY

Some ethnicities have distinct, unique nasal characteristics. Like any other rhinoplasty procedure, the goal is to reshape and refine the nose while minimizing any trauma and possibility of scarring. The changes may be subtle or dramatic, depending on the needs and desires of the patient. What's most important for me and for my patients when doing any rhinoplasty surgery is to alter my patient's nose without diminishing their cultural background or heritage.

ASIAN AND AFRICAN AMERICAN NOSES

Asian and African American noses tend to be characterized by a lower nasal bridge, a broad, flat nasal tip, and a wider frontal view, including the nostrils and bridge. Because this often requires a great deal of cartilage grafting to add to the nose, most of these rhinoplasties are performed through an open approach.

The Nasal Bridge

Many of my Asian and African American rhinoplasty patients want to have their nasal bridge elevated. To do this, I use a cartilage graft, called a dorsal onlay graft, that is created from the septal cartilage or taken from the patient's ear or rib if not enough septal cartilage is present (Figure 38). What's great about using your own cartilage is that your body will incorporate it well because it is not foreign. I prefer not to use implants (silicone, Gore-Tex, or Medpor, to name a few) because they

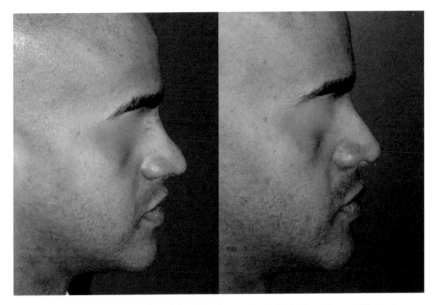

Figure 38: Before (left) and after (right) of a rhinoplasty patient who had cartilage grafting to the nasal bridge because it was too flat and wide.

have a higher rate of infection and can be extruded through the nasal skin.

The Nasal Tip

Many patients that want to have their nasal tip refined feel it lacks projection and is too broad and rounded for their face. Because their nasal tip cartilage is usually weaker while the nasal tip skin is thicker, I often need to use cartilage grafting to refine the tip area and support it using cartilage from inside the nose. In nasal tip surgery for Asian and African Americans, it is important not to use the procedure often performed on Caucasians, where excess nasal tip cartilage is removed, because the nose will pinch (imagine late-career images of Michael Jackson).

The Width of the Nasal Base/Size of the Nostrils

Another common issue with Asian and African American noses involves the excessive width of the nasal base, from one nostril to the other. To narrow the base and nostrils, I do what's called an alar base reduction (Figure 39). Small incisions are made around the sides of the nostrils, and extra skin is removed from the nostrils by making an incision in the crease of the nostril where it meets the cheek. Because the incision is well hidden, the incision lines heal well and are not noticeable. This change is usually subtle and the nose maintains its ethnic character, just without wide nostrils (Figure 40).

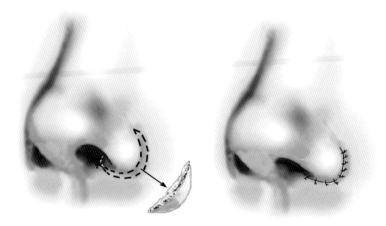

Figure 39: Illustration of the incisions for a nostril reduction surgery called an alar base reduction. The incision is well hidden in the natural groove between the nose and cheek.

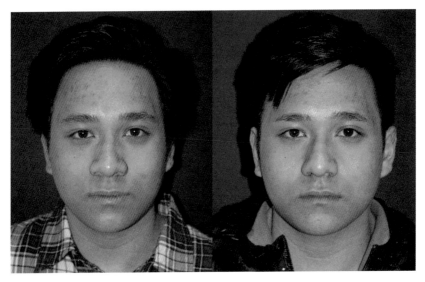

Figure 40: Before (left) and after (right) of a patient who had an alar base reduction, creating a narrower nasal width.

Latino, Hispanic, and Middle Eastern Noses

While some of my Latino, Hispanic, and Middle Eastern patients have the same facial structures as Caucasians, others have slightly different nasal characteristics. One of these different traits is a droopy or hooked nasal tip that can present some challenges when doing tip refinement. If the tip is slightly more hooked or droopy, I do what is called a tongue-and-groove maneuver that helps lift it up. Accessed through an incision on the inside of the nose, the medial crura is sutured to the nasal septum to lift and support the tip (Figure 41). This procedure can be done in isolation, without any other surgery to the rest of the nose, in just thirty minutes under local anesthesia (almost like a visit to the dentist).

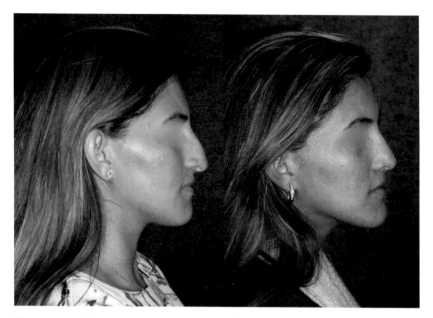

Figure 41: Before (left) and after (right) of a Hispanic patient who had a rhinoplasty with a drooping nasal tip that was lifted using a tongue-and-groove technique.

RHINOPLASTY FOR MEN

Rhinoplasty for men is different than for women, so it's especially important to find a surgeon with a lot of experience on male noses. The aesthetics of the male nose are different from those of the female nose. Men generally strive for a more prominent, powerful nose with distinctive features. Ideally, the nasal tip should be less rotated so that the angle between the upper lip and nose falls around 90 degrees; for women, an angle of 105 degrees is more ideal.

Women who have nose jobs usually want a bridge that is more concave or gently sloped and a refined tip. For men, on the other hand, less is more. I tell them that they really need to *under*-do it. For Caucasians, this means that they rarely want to do anything but straighten the bridge and remove any droopiness of the tip—but even that has to be done very conservatively so as not to feminize the nose. Because there is less aggressive work on the tip, a closed rhinoplasty approach can usually be performed.

In addition, I often tell my male patients *not* to get rid of all of their nasal hump, or anything else that makes their nose distinctive. Even stereotypically handsome, iconic male faces have somewhat bigger noses than normal—think Paul Newman and Tom Cruise with their Roman noses, Jon Hamm with his aquiline nose, and even Liam Neeson with his Irish boxer's nose. For men who already have uniquely structured noses, de-emphasizing it too much can change the balance of

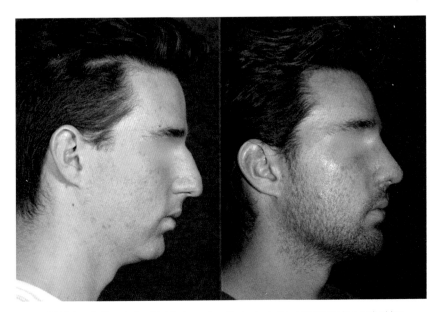

Figure 42: Before (left) and after (right) of a male patient who had a rhinoplasty. In a male rhinoplasty, the bridge should not be overly reduced, creating a strong masculine profile, and the tip should be refined but not overly reduced to avoid feminizing the appearance of the face. He had a chin augmentation with a chin implant at the same time.

their face, and not for the better. It's not about trying to create a perfectly shaped nose. Rather, the goal of rhinoplasty for men is about creating a masculine contour for the face (Figure 42).

BOTCHED RHINOPLASTY: WHAT CAN GO WRONG AND HOW TO FIX IT

The unfortunate truth about rhinoplasty is that somewhere between 10 and 15 percent of the surgeries performed in the United States require revision[2]—the patient is either very unhappy with the results, or there are post-surgery breathing problems. That number is way too high! But that's because a nose can be made too small, the tip can be turned up too much (the classic example being a "piggy nose," where you can see into the nostrils), the bridge can be over-reduced, asymmetry can develop, and the nasal tip or bridge can twist or collapse. Another common problem after rhinoplasty is a bump on the bridge toward the tip, called a polybeak deformity because it makes the nose look like the beak of a bird.

Before you can address any of these problems, you need to wait a complete year after your initial procedure. Sometimes, revision surgery actually isn't needed, and filler can be a welcome alternative to undergoing a more complex surgical redo. This is especially true if the imperfections after surgery are minor (such as small depressions in areas around the tip and bridge). Though the results will be temporary, in many cases it's better to use filler than to deal with more surgery, creating more scar tissue.

For bigger problems, though, revision surgery is the only option. Revision rhinoplasty surgery is usually best performed through an open approach, as it allows the surgeon more access to deal with scar tissue and cartilage distorted by prior surgery. If too much cartilage has been removed, the solution is cartilage grafting (Figure 43). Skull bone, called calvarial bone, may be required in very difficult cases, such as a completely collapsed nose called a saddle nose. Bear in mind that whenever tissues are transplanted to the nose, your recovery will take longer, as your body has to grow into them. Revision rhinoplasty surgery takes more time in the operating room, as well as for post-operative swelling to go down, than after the first surgery. Expect more visits to your doctor to monitor healing and know that sometimes a cortisone shot is necessary to reduce scar formation around the cartilages.

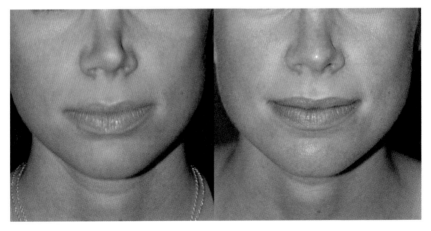

Figure 43: Before (left) and after (right) of a female revision rhinoplasty patient. The pinching of the nasal tip during the prior surgery (performed elsewhere) was created by removing too much cartilage. Reconstruction and shape were accomplished using septal cartilage grafting to the tip during the surgery.

What to Expect After Rhinoplasty Surgery

Rhinoplasties are almost always done on an outpatient basis, with either local or twilight anesthesia. Generally speaking, it takes a few months for the swelling to go down after a rhinoplasty. In the beginning, this is a blessing; your nose was bigger and then it was made smaller, and it swells after surgery. As a result, it doesn't look drastically different at first, so it is easy to fly under the radar. Any swelling of the bridge goes down more quickly than swelling of the tip. It can take a full year to see all of the definition created for the tip after an open rhinoplasty surgery. This tip swelling will resolve more quickly after a closed rhinoplasty.

For the first day or two, there will be a small piece of gauze taped under your nose to help catch excess blood and fluids that try to escape. You will feel congested for the first few days from the swelling inside your nose, but I do not pack the nose, so that there is less pressure. There will be a cast covering your nose, which will remain on for the first week. In many cases, some bruising and swelling will occur, but it is minimal and is usually resolved within a few days. During this time, you should avoid all aerobic physical activity and get as much rest as possible. Keep your head elevated on a few pillows when sleeping or lying down to help prevent swelling. Avoid blowing your nose and wearing glasses for the first four weeks. If you need them for your vision, try to attach the glasses to your forehead using tape, or position a small foam between your nose and the frame of the glasses. Stay out of the sun. Wear hats and use sunscreen, because any sun damage will slow up the healing process and increase swelling.

Try to take the initial post-procedure week off from work or school so when the cast comes off there is minimal or no bruising, and the swelling is not noticeable. Your surgeon will remove the hard cast after one week and do a thorough examination to see how your healing is progressing.

Perhaps more than any other procedure, rhinoplasty requires heavy collaboration between doctor and patient. You'll have to work together to define what you're looking for and to establish how to get it. Before choosing a doctor, be sure to read and follow all of the steps outlined in Chapter 3, focusing especially on how comfortable you feel around your surgeon.

Finally, remember that everyone's face is different. While the nose is an important feature, it must also fit seamlessly into the landscape of the face—it's this balance, or belonging, rather than any shape or size or semblance, that makes a nose "perfect."

---

1 "Plastic Surgery Nightmares," *Us Weekly*, April 2, 2015, https://www.usmagazine.com/stylish/pictures/plastic-surgery-nightmares-2009188/38167/.

2 Keith C. Neaman et al., "Cosmetic Rhinoplasty: Revision Rates Revisited," *Aesthetic Surgery Journal* 33, no. 1 (2013), 31–37, https://academic.oup.com/asj/article/33/1/31/210401.

8 Do Your Lips a Service

Full lips are a symbol of youth, beauty, and sex appeal, which is why, not surprisingly, so many people in the public eye feel the need to have their own lips enhanced. Kylie Jenner wasn't the first celebrity to suddenly appear on our screens with boldly enhanced lips, even if she was the first to get millions of young girls to try to imitate her. Angelina Jolie, Scarlett Johansson, Julia Roberts, Kerry Washington, Megan Fox, not to mention a slew of supermodels, all have particularly pouty, sexy lips, and were on the scene long before Jenner. But over time, I've gotten more and more requests for lip augmentation from patients who are seemingly younger every year—meaning they still have well-defined and full lips. Interestingly, as we will discuss in this chapter, even women in their forties, fifties, and beyond are also adopting this new aesthetic and requesting lip augmentation at record numbers in my practice.

Lip augmentation is also one of the most visible trends in the West Coast style, and when done well, it can look wonderful, especially for those who have naturally thin lips and despaired as they got even thinner with age. Like anything else, regardless if West Coast *or* East Coast style, people can take augmentation too far. There *are* ways to get the fuller lips you crave without looking overdone or unnatural. Results can look completely authentic. It's not about size so much as it is about proportion—but as a reader of this book, you already knew that.

Interestingly, there are some patients who were born with lips that are disproportionately large. Either both the upper and lower lips overwhelm the face, or the upper or lower lip is too big for its counterpart. For these patients, creating balance is as important to their overall beauty as is augmenting smaller lips. This chapter will discuss all of these concepts in depth, along with the nonsurgical and surgical ways of achieving your lip goals.

Natural Lip Aesthetics: The Importance of Proportion

Many of my clients are afraid of lip augmentation, since they see so many examples of "trout pout" or "duck lips" results gone horribly wrong. Ideally, even if one has full, beautiful lips, the upper lip should be smaller than the lower lip (according to the golden ratio, by a factor of 1.618—see Chapter 2). However, some lip augmentations cause that proportion to become reversed, with the upper lip becoming too big and duck bill–like. As the upper lip become overfilled, the peaks of the natural cupid's bow are lost, resulting in an unnatural lip that goes straight across and looks unappealingly like a filled sausage.

Similarly, the distance from the peaks of the cupid's bow to the corners of the mouth should be 1.618 times the distance between the points of the center of the lip. This is true for people of all ethnicities. Even if you want your lips to be more voluptuous and luscious, if these proportions are respected, augmentation will leave your lips looking beautiful and undistorted.

What Happens to Your Lips as You Age

Considering the contemporary focus on fuller lips, it is no wonder that even my middle-aged and older patients are seeking lip augmentation. As we age, our lips lose their fullness, which makes them appear older. The graceful cupid's bow of the upper lip begins to flatten. They go from being full like a grape to deflated like a raisin. There is also an amount of wrinkling that occurs as this volume is lost. The lips descend, increasing the distance between the nose and the upper lip, and they hang over the upper teeth. A lack of tooth show can be associated with a loss of sexuality or sensuality (the aesthetic ideal involves a little bit of tooth show when relaxed lips are parted). Resulting changes in the proportions of your facial features can leave your nasal tip or jawline looking a bit too large for your face. A shorter upper lip, on the other hand, results in a more youthful face because it restores balance. It makes the whole face look a little bit smaller and more petite.

Nonsurgical Lip Procedures

According to the American Academy of Facial Plastic and Reconstructive Surgery, lip augmentation using injectable fillers is one of the most common facial plastic procedures performed today.[1] In fact, the number of people coming to my office for lip procedures has increased more than for any other facial procedure.

Lip fillers are a great option if you want fuller lips, whether yours have thinned out due to aging or because they've been naturally thin since birth; or if you want to reshape lips that might be disproportionate in some way, such as those that naturally turn downward; or if you want to better define the cupid's bow and/or to minimize any lipstick-bleed lines.

TEMPORARY FILLERS

The most common injectable fillers used for lips are hyaluronic acid–based fillers like the Restylane and Juvederm families of products. I say family because there are many different formulations of each, such as Restylane Silk, Restylane Defyne, Juvederm Volbella, and Juvederm Vollure. These companies have made many subtypes, and different practitioners have different preferences, depending on the properties they're seeking for a particular patient or procedure. There is no perfect hyaluronic filler and they all do a great job; it just depends on the doctor's preference. All temporary lip fillers will last only four to six months. Because the lips move so much, the filler tends to degrade faster than when it is injected in the cheeks, eyelids, or nose.

As I stated previously, many of my clients who are considering lip augmentation are afraid of undergoing the procedure because of all the exaggerated outcomes they see. More traditional techniques can create the overtly overfilled lip they dread, but newer, more evolved techniques can avoid this. I allay their fears by explaining that I will under-do the treatment and allow them to see what I am doing with a mirror, step by step, so that they can be reassured that I am not over-injecting. I explain that if they decide that they do not like the results, I can inject an enzyme called hyaluronidase to dissolve the material away in twenty-four hours.

The traditional lip filler technique involves injecting the filler into the lip (or vermillion) border and filling the lip as you withdraw the needle. This makes the lip one shape throughout and blunts the natural contours of the lip and cupid's bow. The lip then looks unnatural, overstuffed.

Instead of this "old" technique, I use the classification system I developed for placement of fillers, which allows me to precisely target, with more natural results, fifteen different anatomical zones on the lips (Figure 44).[2] As everyone's lips are different, in one patient I may need to inject only three zones, and in another ten zones, to attain the correct size and proportional shape. This allows me to create custom lips for my Park Avenue patients that are enviably full but never plastic-looking

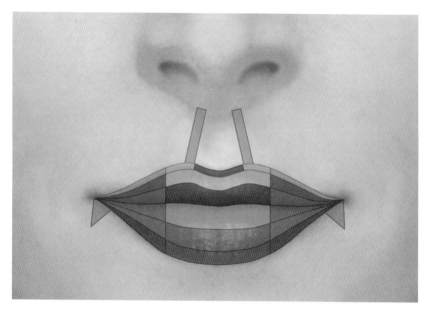

Figure 44: Illustration demonstrating fifteen different anatomic zones used to direct lip augmentation with injectable fillers. These zones are injected differentially to create natural-appearing customized lips and avoid an overfilled "trout pout."

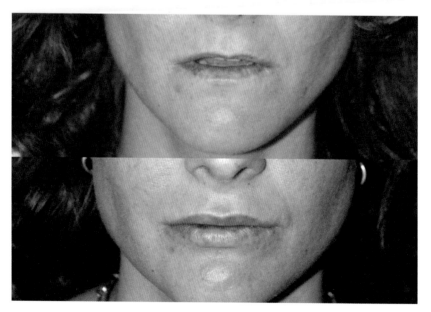

Figure 45: Before (top) and after (bottom) of a patient who had a lip augmentation with injectable hyaluronic acid to create fuller lips. Notice the natural smooth contours.

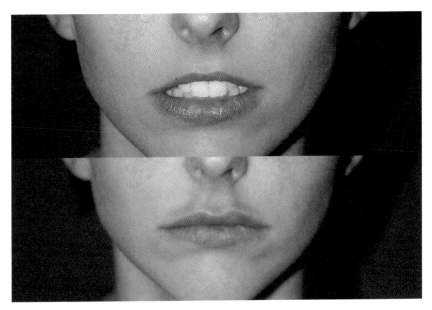

Figure 46: Before (top) and after (bottom) of a patient who desired a "French lips" lip augmentation with injectable hyaluronic acid to create a poutier, more stylized lip.

(Figure 45). Many of my patients request what I call "French lips," a more voluptuous yet still balanced lip. I use Restylane or Juvederm injections to sculpt the lips so that the central portion of the upper lip is pouty and the inside of the lip is rolled out (Figure 46). It gives a lovely and natural shape to the lips.

PERMANENT LIP INJECTIONS

While most lip injections are temporary, silicone injections are permanent. Silicone is not FDA-approved for use in the lips, and I don't use it. There is a small but real risk that the lip can react negatively to the silicone and create nodules and reactive tissue called granulomas, causing lumpiness and irregularities, even when it is injected perfectly. Delayed reactions can occur, even ten years after it is injected. There is also a risk that, as you age and the lips thin, the silicone can start to show through as an unsightly roll in the lip. I have performed hundreds of surgeries to re-contour the lips of patients who had silicone injections with good doctors. It is not the technique that is the problem; it is the material. I make an incision line inside the lip to access the material and re-contour it (Figure 47). For this reason, I will not inject silicone, but after explaining these problems to patients who then decide they still want it, I refer them to one of my dermatology colleagues practicing in New York who has injected tens of thousands of lips using silicone and who is the best in the business at it.

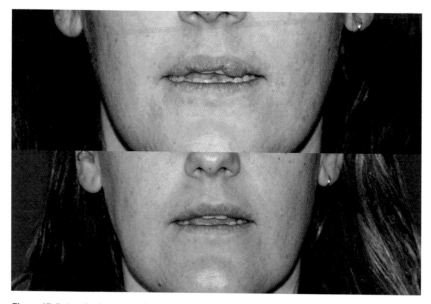

Figure 47: Before (top) and after (bottom) of a patient who had corrective plastic surgery from a prior lip augmentation with permanent silicone injection (performed elsewhere) that created nodules (granulomas) and distortion. Corrective surgery requires incisions inside the lips to remove the material and smooth these contours.

Surgical Lip Procedures

One of the most common reasons I see patients for a surgical lip augmentation consultation is filler fatigue; after many years of lip augmentation with temporary fillers, many patients want a more permanent solution. The second most common reason is when lip injections do not achieve a patient's desired goal. Other surgical procedures include different lip lifts that treat a long upper lip (which many people have even in their youth), a hanging upper lip (which happens as we age), and lip reduction, to bring disproportionately large lips into harmony with the rest of the face.

LIP AUGMENTATION SURGERIES

For All Ethnicities

Theoretically permanent, fat transfer, first discussed back in Chapter 5, can also be used to treat lips. This procedure involves suctioning your own body fat from the abdomen or thighs and transferring it into the lips. I will place the fat in the same anatomic subunits described in Figure 44 (page 190). While fat grafting seems like a good idea because it uses your own body tissue, because the lips move, there is a lower "take rate" than there is with fat grafting elsewhere in the face; at least half the time, the fat grafting reabsorbs completely. I explain this to patients and often suggest they try some other surgical treatment (to be described) that is more permanent. If I am doing a fat transfer for the cheeks and the patient also wants their lips injected, we have extra fat available. If it takes, it is a bonus—but if not, their cheeks have been treated, and we'll pursue a different procedure for the lips.

There are better options that use tissue from your own body to augment the lips. One is called a dermal fat graft, where a combination of the deep portion of your skin and fat are harvested together. This requires an incision that is usually placed above your bikini line (if you have had a C-section, you can use this old incision). Once this strip of tissue is removed from the abdomen, it is placed in the upper and lower lips via a small cut in the inside corner of the mouth that is not visible. The grafts can be custom designed to fulfill your desire for shape, and because it is a tissue graft and not suctioned fat, the take rates are very high.

Because lips become thinner as we age, it is very common for me to do this procedure on patients who are getting a facelift to rejuvenate their overall look. What is different in the case of a combined facelift and lip tissue graft is that we can borrow from some of the redundant loose muscle in the face while inside of it and no additional incisions are required to get the tissue to transfer. The muscle we use is called the superficial musculo aponeurotic system, and this technique is called an SMAS graft (Figure 48).

Some doctors use tubes of hard silicone and place them through the same small incisions. Not only do I not like to use plastic in the lips, but I also have taken them out of many patients who complain that they feel hard and unnatural, even though they look great. It would make sense that a plastic rod in your lip would feel strange, and I do not suggest it.

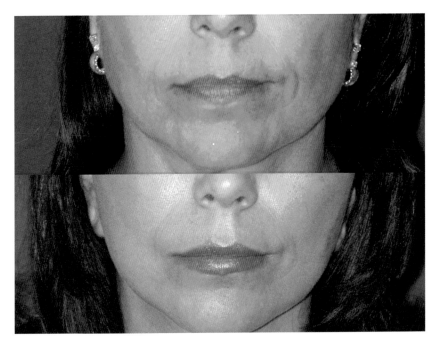

Figure 48: Before (top) and after (bottom) of a patient who had an SMAS lip augmentation, where muscles from the face are transferred to the lips with a small incision in the corner of the mouth. This creates a permanent lip augmentation that does not require repeated injections with filler that dissolves away.

Another technique is a procedure called a V-to-Y lip augmentation, which creates permanent, voluptuous lips that are more stylized. This is for my patients who want lips like Angelina Jolie, with the outer corner of the lips turned out and the lip full and pouty. This procedure is not requested by many of my East Coast patients, but patients from the West Coast will fly in for this surgery because very few surgeons in this country do it. V-to-Y surgery uses incisions on the inside of the lips; then, the lip is rolled from the inside out, making it pouty and full. Because the incisions are on the inside of the lips, there are no visible scars (Figure 49). I've performed

A
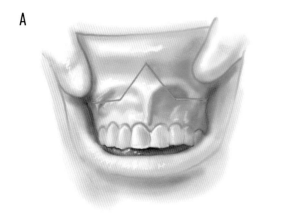

B
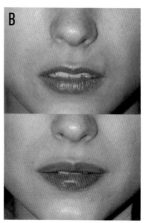

Figure 49: A) Incisions for a V-to-Y lip augmentation. B) Before (top) and after (bottom) of a patient who had a V-to-Y lip augmentation. Rolling the lips from the inside out creates fuller, "poutier" lips such as Angelina Jolie's.

studies on this technique, which can be adjusted so that lips are augmented more subtly or more aggressively (as in cases of very thin lips).[3] The upper and lower lips can also be augmented differently, and I can increase the curvature of the cupid's bow as well. A big procedure with a longer recovery, it takes, on average, three weeks or more for recovery, because the lips swell a lot. Even though I am one of the few surgeons who perform it, it's not one of my most common surgeries, because it addresses a very specific desire for more exaggerated lips.

LIP LIFTS

Lip lifts are some of my favorite procedures to perform, since they illustrate how such a small procedure can have such a large impact on the overall beauty of the face. A lip lift elevates the lip to reveal a broader smile and shorten the distance between the nose and the upper lip. It exposes more of the upper teeth at rest. And for those with a very thin upper lip, it gives fullness to the upper lip and can bring it to a better aesthetic proportion with the lower lip. The end result is a permanent lip augmentation. The operation can be tailored to elevate different sections of the lip along the central cupid's bow to make them shapelier. Performing these surgeries on older patients can lift the visual perspective of the face and can trick the eye into thinking an entire facelift has been done. This subtle alteration makes people look years younger and rejuvenated.

There are four main types of lip lifts, all done through hidden incisions along anatomic borders: bullhorn, gull wing, Italian, and corner. The most common is the bullhorn (subnasal) lip lift. During this procedure, an incision in the shape of a bull's horns is made just beneath your nose. A tiny strip of skin and tissue is removed, the muscle is tightened, and the upper lip is raised to its new position. Your scar is virtually undetectable, as it is hidden in the curves of your nose. This procedure can also be customized to elevate the central lip or corners of the lip. I determine where to place the lip by having the patient lift the upper lip with their fingers to the preferred position, paying attention to how much the teeth show. A subtler lip lift leaves approximately 13 to 14 millimeters between the lip and nose, or 10 to 12 millimeters with a more stylized lip lift (Figure 50).

A gull wing lift removes a strip of skin above the border of your upper lip. The cutout is M-shaped to advance the border

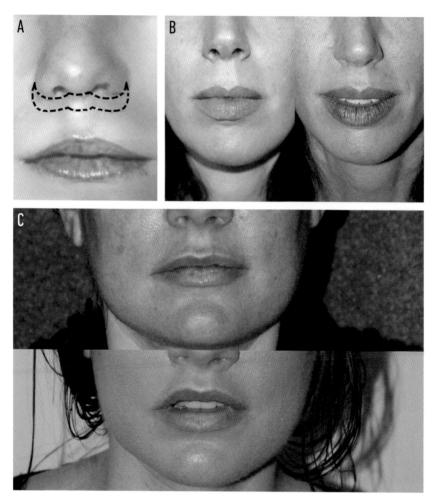

Figure 50: A) Incisions for a "bullhorn" upper lip lift. B) Before (left) and after (right) of a patient who had a bullhorn upper lip lift with a subtler result. C) Before (top) and after (bottom) of a patient who had a bullhorn upper lip lift with a poutier, more stylized result.

of your upper lip. The incision is made where the pink part of your upper lip meets the skin above it. This lip lift leaves a more visible scar, and as a result I rarely do this procedure. It is most effective in patients who are older and have fairly thin skin. Its real utility is to advance the border of the lip that flattens more significantly with age. I would never do this surgery on a patient younger than sixty years old (Figure 51).

The Italian lip lift is an alternative to a bullhorn lip lift. For those who need less of a lift, the incisions can be modified. The Italian lip lift requires two separate incisions (smaller than that used in a bullhorn lift) that are hidden beneath each nostril. Skin is removed, and the right and left sides of the lip are each separately lifted by closing the wound and reducing the distance between the lip and nose (Figure 52).

Lastly, there is the corner lip lift. Corner lip lifts are for people who have lips that are naturally turned down at the corners, making them look sad or discouraged. They can also improve grooves at the corner of the mouth that drift down toward the chin, often referred to as drool grooves. The incisions are made at the outer corners where the upper and lower

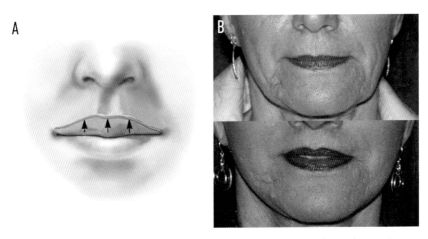

Figure 51: A) Incisions for a "gull wing" upper lip lift. B) Before (top) and after (bottom) of a patient who had a gull wing upper lip lift. This procedure is used less commonly and for more aged upper lips.

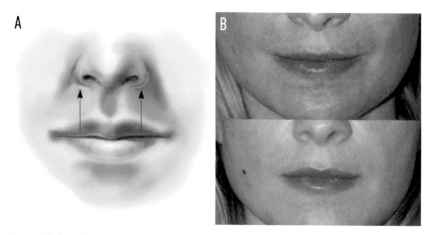

Figure 52: A) Incisions for an Italian upper lip lift. B) Before (top) and after (bottom) of a patient who had an Italian upper lip lift. This procedure has smaller incisions and is used when less of a lift is necessary.

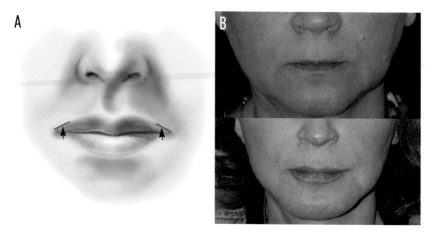

Figure 53: A) Incisions for a corner lip lift. B) Before (top) and after (bottom) of a patient who had a corner lip lift. This procedure is used on older patients with a downturned mouth with deep marionette lines.

lips meet. A small triangular area of skin is removed so that the lips turn up slightly in a more youthful manner. If the grooves are deep and prominent, surgery may not provide 100 percent correction, but there is major improvement (Figure 53).

LIP PROCEDURES FOR MEN

Unless a man has unusually thin, ribbon-like lips, I'm not a big fan of manipulating male lips. The results can look peculiar or feminizing. If men do want larger lips, they're much better off using temporary hyaluronic acid fillers so the results can be reversed.

BOTCHED LIP PROCEDURES: WHAT CAN GO WRONG AND HOW TO FIX IT

One potential problem with lip augmentation occurs with fat grafting. Doctors who use fat often overfill the lips because they assume some of the fat will reabsorb, but if all the fat remains, or if only some of it is absorbed, this can leave the lips too large. To correct this, at first an attempt is made to dissolve the fat with a shot of a cortisone-like medicine called Kenalog. If this doesn't work, liposuction is attempted with a thin microcannula, which is inserted under the lip skin like a needle. If this fails, the only option left is a lip reduction, as shown in the procedure used in Figure 47 on page 192. The same correction techniques apply for an overdone dermal fat graft or SMAS lip graft (Figure 54).

Complications can also result from lip implants made of silicone. If the implant shifts or extrudes, removal through an incision inside the lip is advisable; then, after the lips heal, most doctors repeat the lip augmentation with tissue from your own body.

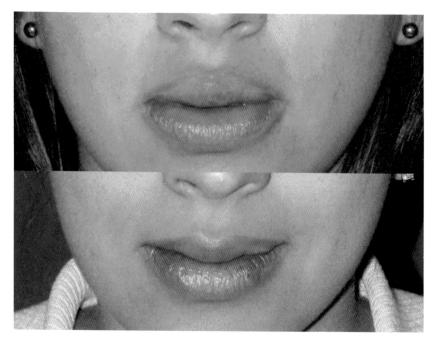

Figure 54: Before (top) and after (bottom) of a patient who had a corrective lip reduction after having excessive fat grafting to the lips (performed elsewhere), to create a more natural proportion.

What to Expect After Lip Surgery

Lip procedures are almost always done on an outpatient basis, under local anesthesia. Most of them take no longer than forty-five minutes to an hour. Recovery from most lip lifts takes about five to seven days. The exception is the V-to-Y lip enhancement, which takes four to six weeks to heal. I tell all of my lip procedure patients to avoid kissing for three weeks.

The newfound popularity of lip enhancement and augmentation procedures perfectly exemplifies how profoundly beauty trends can affect the decisions of plastic surgery patients. The aesthetics of facial beauty are always in flux and, as mentioned in Part I, differ from culture to culture. But when deliberating about whether or not to go under the knife, reflect on the influences behind your decision to have a surgical procedure. Trends are fleeting—do you want to change your face permanently to reflect a flash-in-the-pan fashion? Luckily, there are a number of beautifully effective temporary procedures available for lips. If you are going the permanent route, however, take some time to think about how you'll feel about your new look five, ten, fifteen years from now. As with any surgery, preparation is key.

---

1 "Facial Plastic Trends Reported; Filler Injections Are Up," *Facial Plastic Surgery Today* 25, no. 2 (2011), https://www.aafprs.org/patient/fps_today/vol25/02/pg1.html.

2 Andrew A. Jacono, "A New Classification of Lip Zones to Customize Injectable Lip Augmentation," *Archives of Facial Plastic Surgery* 10, no. 1 (2008), 25–29, doi: 10.1001/archfaci.10.1.25, https://www.ncbi.nlm.nih.gov/pubmed/18209119.

3 Andrew A. Jacono and Vito C. Quatela, "Quantitative Analysis of Lip Appearance after V-Y Lip Augmentation," *Archives of Facial Plastic Surgery* 6, no. 3 (2004), 172–177, doi: 10.1001/archfaci.6.3.172, https://www.ncbi.nlm.nih.gov/pubmed/15148125.

9 Your Face as Sculpture

Shaping Cheeks, Chins, Ears, and Hairlines

Often, men and women come to my office requesting to modify a specific facial feature. They might want higher cheekbones, a smaller chin, fewer wrinkles. Or they might want to augment a weak chin that makes their face look imbalanced.

But others tell me, "I don't look like myself anymore. Why has my face changed so much?" The answer often lies in the features that frame our face, including our cheeks and chin. They're not pointing to wrinkles, lines, or age spots. They're pointing to structural changes that gradually take place all over their faces with time. These changes occur from the tops of our heads to the bottoms of our chins. While we will cover aging changes that occur along the jawline and neck in Chapter 10 and have already discussed changes in the center of the face, including the nose and lips, in Chapters 7 and 8, this chapter will focus on the features of our face that are in the periphery. Even our ears change with age! And while we don't often think of our hair as a structural feature, it is the painting on the frame, and a thin or recessed hairline will not allow all the other features of our face to shine through. Hairline issues are not just experienced by men; many women also struggle with female pattern balding.

Let's take a look at the nonsurgical and surgical procedures you can consider that will sculpt your face and bring back its youthful contours.

Your Facial Skeletal Structure

The most defining structural features of the facial frame are the cheekbones and the chin. There is a wide variety of "beautiful" cheek shapes and structures, and there is no ideal cheek shape or size. It is true, however, that there are facial skeletal features that are considered to be more feminine and attractive. This is related to human biology: Anthropometric studies have shown that women with high levels of estrogen, and thus high reproductive potential, have higher cheekbones. This makes them more attractive to the opposite sex. While not germane to this chapter, it is also why men are traditionally more attracted to women with larger lips and breasts and wider hips.

One of the strongest characteristics of youth is fullness of the cheeks—those pinchable apple cheeks with a soft, oval volume—indicating an abundance of healthy soft tissues and fat under the skin. Beautiful cheeks are defined by their height and volume; my patients often tell me that they want high, well-defined cheekbones coupled with a natural roundness. Flat cheekbones can make a large nose look larger and a receding chin look smaller. The cheekbones, in fact, are largely responsible for defining your face, highlighting your eyes, and adding balance to your features. In Chapter 2, we discussed a guideline using the golden ratio to define the ideal size and shape of the cheek, but that does not mean that we should transpose this specifically on every face. Balancing the cheeks with all the other facial features is the true artistry of plastic surgery.

Sometimes the cheeks can be too full and round—what patients call "chipmunk cheeks," "chubby cheeks," or even "baby-faced cheeks." This happens when you have excess buccal fat pads, located in the lower portion of the cheeks near the corner of the mouth, which make your cheeks look plumper when you want them to look sculpted. Because the size and location of the fat pads is genetically determined, they can't be reduced by diet or exercise. The solution is to have a cheek reduction, using a technique called a buccal fat pad removal, which I will discuss in this chapter. This technique will slim the cheeks, creating more defined cheekbones.

A recessed or large chin also creates an imbalance in overall facial harmony. Interestingly, chin augmentation can improve the appearance of the nose, making it look smaller, so many people who think they need a nose job actually don't after they make their chin a little bit bigger. If a woman's chin is too projected, it can be masculinizing to the appearance, which is why we perform chin reduction surgery. On the contrary, a stronger chin in men is desirable and projects a masculine, in-charge appearance. Believe it or not, one study of the top fifty Fortune 500 companies shows that 90 percent of CEOs had prominent chins, compared to 40 percent of the rest of the United States population.[1] We tend to have more confidence in the ability of those who have this facial feature.

What Happens to Your Facial Structure as You Age

As we age, our faces go from being more heart-shaped to square-shaped. You can almost think of the young cheek like a plush grape. As the grape loses volume and dehydrates, it becomes a raisin with nothing more than a deflated shell. The distance between the cheeks and the distance between the lower face along the jawline become equal.

These changes take place due to the distribution of the under-lying facial fatty tissue; some of the facial fat reduces with age (a process called atrophy) and some of the fat actually droops due to gravity. Re-volumizing the cheeks either nonsurgically or surgically will lift them up like a reinflated balloon and reestablish the more youthful heart shape.

Unfortunately, if you had smaller, flatter cheekbones or a small, receding chin in your youth, your face will age more rapidly. Your cheek and chin bones act as a scaffolding for your facial soft tissues. A larger skeletal structure will hold up the face and age better than a face with less structure. When we are older, adding a chin implant will support and improve jowling along the neck and jawline, and adding a cheek implant will lift drooping cheeks.

Nonsurgical Cheek and Chin Augmentation

There are two noninvasive ways to augment the facial skeleton: with injectable fillers and with fat transfer from your own body. The easiest and least invasive way to reshape your face is with injectable fillers, such as hyaluronic acid fillers. Autologous fat transfer does not require open surgery, but it is more invasive than just opening a package of filler. You must harvest the fat and then inject it into the face with cannulas. Chapter 5 describes in detail the different available fillers and their qualities, but, as a brief review, my favorites are Voluma and Restylane Lyft because these hyaluronic acid gels have a more supportive nature than others. My Park Avenue patients want to fly under the radar. They do not like the West Coast style's aesthetic of an overfilled cheek with the upper, middle, and lower cheek on either side of the nose filled. Overfilling can cause people to look almost simian or monkey-like—the cheeks might not be as droopy, but they certainly don't look beautiful. To avoid this, the site of the injection makes all the difference. The injections should be made deeply, over the cheekbones, which supports the face more than if they were just injected superficially into the skin or muscles.

As you know, fat transfer involves suctioning out fat from the abdomen, flanks, or thighs, and then injecting it into the face. I use the same placement as with temporary fillers. The problem with fat, as discussed at greater length in Chapter 5, is that I can never predict how much will stick. While fat can be permanent in 60 percent of transfer cases, for those looking for a guaranteed, permanent outcome, the best option is a customized cheek implant.

The same fillers and fat techniques are used for the chin. A general guideline used by plastic surgeons to determine the ideal projection and size of the chin involves taking a photograph of the patient's face in profile and drawing a vertical line from the point where the nose and lip meet straight down (Figure 55). If the chin falls behind that line, the chin is considered to be small or weak, and if it is in front of this line, it is considered excessive. For women, I feel that the chin should

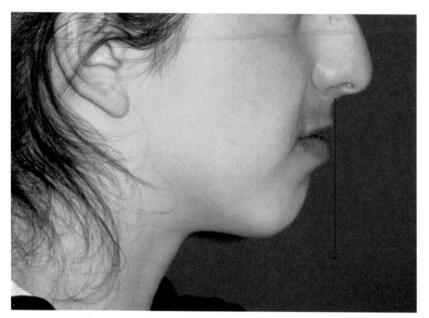

Figure 55: To determine if a chin has proper aesthetic balance with the face, plastic surgeons draw a vertical line down from the meeting point of the upper lip and nose. If the chin is behind the line, it is considered proportionally small; if in front of the line, too large.

be a less prominent feature and should usually fall 1 to 2 millimeters behind this line, to avoid looking too structural or masculine. I inject the filler or fat so that the most projected area of the chin comes to the point of a soft oval. In men, it is more desirable for the chin to be slightly forward of this line, and the chin should be squarer, with two prominent points to the right and left of the midline. I have never had a male patient who underwent chin augmentation and asked for it to be smaller. They always want it a little bigger, which we can accomplish with another injection session.

If you feel like your cheeks or chin are too big, there is no nonsurgical way to reduce them. In this case, surgery is the only option.

Surgical Procedures for Cheeks, Chins, and Jaws

For All Ethnicities

There are two types of surgery you can have to reshape your cheeks, chin, and jaw: implant (which will increase volume) or reduction (which will make the area smaller). Most implant or reduction surgery is done under local or twilight anesthesia, so general surgery is not required.

Cheek implant surgery is performed through an incision made inside the mouth where your upper lip meets your gums. This hidden incision means that there are no visible scars. Then a pocket over the actual cheekbone is created where the implant is placed. The implant is fixed with a titanium screw so that it can never move or become malpositioned. After the

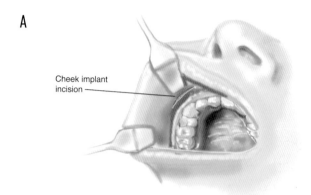

A

Cheek implant
incision

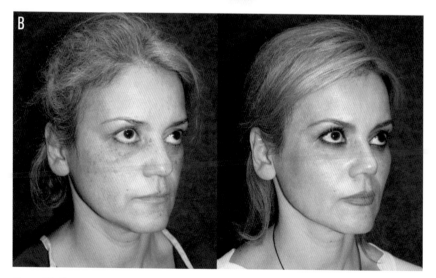

B

Figure 56: A) Incision for a cheek augmentation with cheek implants hidden inside the mouth. B) Before (left) and after (right) of a patient who had a cheek augmentation.

implant is perfectly fitted, the incision is closed, often with one stitch. Supportive tissue eventually forms around the implant after a few weeks, and, once fully healed, the implant feels like your normal underlying bone structure (Figure 56).

Implants can be made of Silastic, Medpor, or Gore-Tex. Silastic is a hard polymer implant material that has been used in hundreds of millions of patients worldwide with the lowest

Bespoke Implants

One of the most amazing technological advances in plastic surgery is the ability to make custom, bespoke implants. To create them, I work with a team of computer engineers. First, my patient has a CT scan. This gives me a three-dimensional computer representation of their skeletal structure. With this data I can create a cheek implant to fit the patient's personal style (Figure 57); it can also address any asymmetries (we all have about a 7 to 15 percent difference in size between the two sides of our face). After the initial modeling, I meet with my patient and we go over the design to make sure that we're on the same page. Once we make final approvals, I render the data and export it to a company called Implant Tech, which takes that computer model and creates a mold for it. The material is made of Silastic. Because they are custom engineered to the

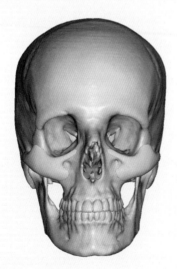

Figure 57: Bespoke facial implants are made by modeling the implants after using a CT scan of facial bones. The implants are custom-made to create the exact proportions desired. This is the best way to make implants—but also the costliest.

patient's existing facial skeleton, they fit on the surface of the cheekbones like a key in a latch. It's a very satisfying process for everyone because each implant is specifically engineered to my patients' desires and anatomies.

Because bespoke implants are expensive, many patients will opt for prefabricated implants. Even though they are not custom, this is not a one-size-fits-all procedure. I will often place many different implant shapes and sizes into the pocket during surgery using sizers (or test implants) to find the best fit for the patient's face before I choose the one I will use. Sometimes I need to further sculpt the implants by hand to make everything balance.

rate of infection and extrusion. The body creates a capsule around these implants so it is easy to remove them or replace them with an implant of a different size if your goals change in the future. Gore-Tex and Medpor are also hard polymers, but the body grows into them. This makes them extremely difficult to modify, so I prefer not to use them. I have had patients come to me to remove Gore-Tex or Medpor implants placed years ago, and they get extremely scarred into place so that it can take several hours to cut through the scar tissue to remove them, resulting in a long recovery and difficulty replacing them with another size or shape if desired by the patient. My advice would be to avoid these implants.

The incision to reduce full or chubby cheeks is made in the same place inside the mouth as with a cheek implant surgery.

A

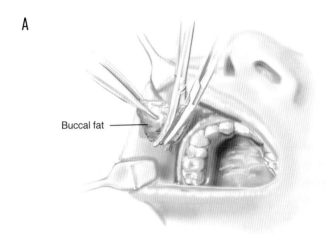

Buccal fat

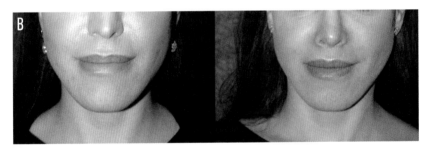

Figure 58: A) Incision for a buccal fat extraction hidden inside the mouth, allowing access for removal of the buccal fat pad. B) Before (left) and after (right) of a buccal fat extraction patient, showing a more defined face after reducing fuller cheeks.

Through this incision, the buccal space, where the buccal fat (which looks like a large walnut in each cheek) lives, is entered. The buccal fat cannot be accessed with a simple liposuction because it exists under the facial muscles and nerves, which could be damaged (Figure 58). The amount of buccal fat removed is how the difference between West Coast and East Coast styles is most evident. Many celebrities have had too much buccal fat removed from their faces, which makes it look like they are sucking their cheeks in; they have too

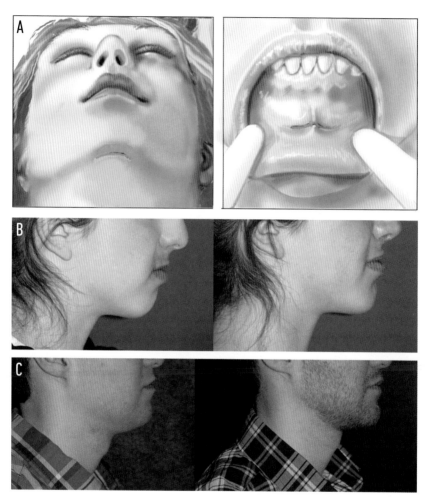

Figure 59: A) Incision options for a chin augmentation: hidden on the inside of the lip or under the chin. Both approaches work, but the external approach has fewer problems with the chin implant moving. B) Before (left) and after (right) of a female patient's chin augmentation with an implant. C) Before (left) and after (right) of a male patient's chin augmentation with an implant. Implants in women should be subtler to look natural. In men, they should be stronger to create a more masculine contour.

much hollowing under their cheekbones, which can produce an unnatural, skeletal effect. For a natural face, it is important to reduce and contour the buccal fat rather than remove it totally. It is a quick and simple procedure.

For patients desiring chin augmentation, the chin implant is inserted through a small incision inside the lower lip or under the chin, which leaves a barely noticeable and well-hidden scar (Figure 59). Although patients may prefer the internal incision, I issue a word of caution against this approach. When placing a chin implant through an incision inside the mouth, a ligament that holds the lip to the chin gets cut. In a small but real percentage of cases, this can lead to a change in the appearance of the lower lip and can affect the appearance of your smile. Also, the implants have a higher rate of shifting and malpositioning with this approach, and, after many years of smiling and expressing your face, the implant can ride up into your mouth, pushing up against your gums. For these reasons, I prefer to make the incision under the chin, but I can and will place it internally as long as the patient understands the risks. The incision under the chin preserves these ligaments and averts these problems. The incision used externally is small, only 1 centimeter, and, hidden under the chin, it heals fantastically well.

Chin reduction surgery is performed through the same incision as that for a chin implant. Again, this procedure is done far more often on women than on men, because a stronger chin and jawline is a more desirable trait in men. Through this incision, I use an ultrasonic-driven bone-reduction instrument to precisely shape, reduce, and contour the chin. Chin reduction surgery can be just as transformative as a chin implant.

Some people have good cheek and chin structure but weak jaws. Jaw implants are also referred to as gonial angle implants because they augment the angle of the jaw (the gonial angle). While gonial implants are common for women and men with small jaws, they can also bring more masculinity and balance to the male face. This does not mean they will masculinize a woman's face when done appropriately; in fact, some iconic women with defined gonial angles and jawlines include Audrey Hepburn and Angelina Jolie. Definition along the jaw creates an elegant contour as it transitions into the neck.

These implants are generally placed through incisions hidden inside the mouth, farther back along the jawline, at the crease where the inside of your lower lips and gums meet (Figure 60). They are then shaped to match the jawline and adhere tightly along that contour. The implant is ultimately held in place with two to three titanium screws. This procedure is repeated on the opposite side. The incision is closed in layers

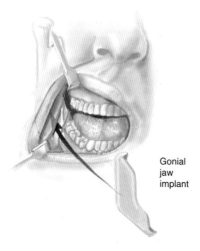

Gonial
jaw
implant

Figure 60: Incision options for a gonial angle or jawline implant are hidden on the inside of the mouth.

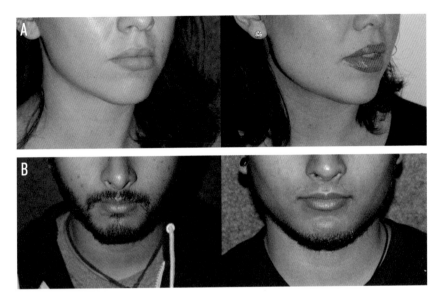

Figure 61: Before (left) and after (right) of gonial angle implants. In women this will give them a defined jawline like Audrey Hepburn; in men a rugged jawline like Brad Pitt. A) Female patient. B) Male patient.

so that there is a watertight seal to keep the oral fluids out of the wound. Insertion of a jaw implant usually takes about one to two hours. Jaw implants are different than chin implants, but people with small jaw angles often have weak chins and could benefit from a simultaneous chin augmentation procedure (Figure 61).

FOREHEAD REJUVENATION

We have already discussed how to lift drooping foreheads and brows in Chapter 6. One area of the forehead that is often overlooked is the temples. As we get older, usually starting in our forties, the temples sink in and become concave, which is called temporal atrophy. Adding volume back to this area can instantly take years off someone's face. The muscle you chew

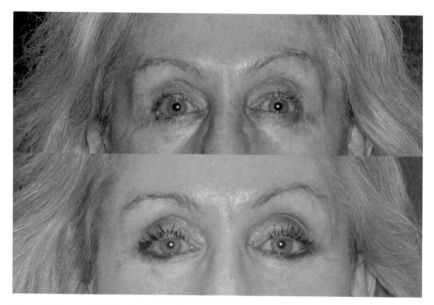

Figure 62: Before (top) and after (bottom) of a patient who had fat grafting to the temples. Additional fat grafting was performed to the upper and lower eyelid hollowing. As we age, the temples and eyes lose volume and become concave.

with, called the temporalis muscle, is located in this area, and is the culprit behind temple hollowing. The injections go on top of this muscle so that the concavity fills in (Figure 62).

Just like with cheeks and chins, I will inject filler or fat in this area, often in combination with augmentation procedures on other parts of the face.

UNIQUE CHARACTERISTICS FOR ASIAN FACIAL RESTRUCTURING

Asian patients have higher rates of buccal fat excess and chubby cheeks, but when they have a consultation with me to discuss facial narrowing, they often don't know that buccal fat is the culprit. Additionally, the cheekbone structure in many Asians is broad and wide. The cheekbones can be re-contoured and made smaller with the same ultrasonic technology used in chin reduction surgery. Since I work through the same hidden incisions used for the buccal fat extraction, it is common for both procedures to be performed at the same time.

Not only can the cheeks appear broad in Asian patients, the lower face can appear wide as well. This is caused by either a wider jawbone, especially at the angle of the jaw, or because the masseter muscles we use to chew are too bulky. The masseter muscles lie over the jaw angles, and you can tell if yours are excessive by biting your teeth together briskly and feeling if the width of the face increases. If bony excess is the primary cause, an ultrasonic bone-reducing device is used to reduce the bone (inserted through the same type of incision required for a gonial angle implant). Unfortunately, there is no surgery that permanently reduces the masseter muscle. Botox injections into the muscles make them flatten, but only last for four to six months. The amount of Botox required for this large muscle is four times what is injected for wrinkles, so the cost is often three to four times that of a simple Botox treatment.

FACIAL RESTRUCTURING FOR MEN

Athletic men often develop hollows at their temples and under the cheekbones that make them look drawn. If they have extremely low body fat percentages, their buccal fat regresses. Adding fillers or fat to these areas can make a man look healthier. These athletic males are a specific subset of men, because generally I do not think that men look good with fillers or fat transfers. Men's faces are supposed to look somewhat rugged and chiseled, and soft cheeks with a lot of replaced volume can be feminizing.

BOTCHED FACIAL STRUCTURE SURGERY: WHAT CAN GO WRONG AND HOW TO FIX IT

Implants that are the wrong size or shape can only be surgically removed. I prefer to use Silastic implants, as you read earlier in this chapter, because they don't cause as much internal scarring and cause fewer infections. The problem with porous polymethylene and Gore-Tex implants is that the body grows into them, causing extensive scarring, which makes them very difficult to remove. In addition, if an implant twists, it requires revision surgery, adjusting the implant and screwing it into the bone to create a stable position.

Buccal fat removal is a permanent procedure, and you want to make sure that your surgeon removes *only* the necessary amount of excess buccal fat to give you the more sculpted and slimming contour you want. The entire fat pad should not ever be removed, as this can create cheeks that are too hollow. Sometimes, I have prospective patients in their teens or twenties who ask for this procedure, even though they don't have particularly round cheeks, because they've read that this can give them an even more sculpted look and higher cheekbones. I tell them that it's not a good idea as they might be very sorry in a decade or so when their facial fat naturally starts to lessen, and that they will start to look prematurely much older and much more haggard. When too much fat has been removed, the best option is replacement with fat grafting.

What to Expect After Facial Structure Surgery

Implant surgery and buccal fat removal have quick recoveries, and many of my patients will only take three days off from work, or do it on a Friday and go back to work Monday. There can be some mild bruising, but if it persists, I instruct my patients to tell friends and colleagues that they just had their wisdom teeth removed if they prefer to keep the procedure to themselves.

Skeletal reduction surgery, when we remove bone, creates more bruising, so one week off work is more appropriate.

Don't Forget About Your Ears

Ears are incredibly distinctive. We all have ears of different sizes and positions within the framework of our facial features. The ears are to the face as earrings are to the ears themselves. Because they are worn on the face like jewelry, they draw a lot of attention to themselves.

Protruding ears can make both children and adults self-conscious and miserable, especially if they've been teased or bullied. Many men and women will wear long hair to hide their ears and refuse to put their hair up in a baseball cap or ponytail in fear of exposing them. As you age, gravity is no more kind to your earlobes than it is to the rest of your face and body. Because the lobes are made only of skin and fibro-fatty tissue, they can get very long and droopy—making your entire ear look larger. For many women, the earlobes are not really noticed unless they like to wear earrings. The weight of heavier earrings can cause the earlobe to stretch and lengthen even more. Earlobes also become thin and shriveled with age, which leaves them marked with unsightly folds and creases.

Nonsurgical Ear Procedures

When earlobes become stretched out, injecting them with hyaluronic acid filler will stiffen and lift them slightly, just like blowing up a balloon. This approach also helps shriveled earlobes, and narrow, stretched earlobe holes that enlarge with age and earring use. I prefer Restylane, as I do in nonsurgical rhinoplasty, because Restylane is one of the most supportive fillers and will lift the earlobes higher than others. Because the earlobes do not move at all, fillers can last up to two years in this location. Fat grafting can also be attempted for more permanent correction.

Surgical Ear Procedures

For All Ethnicities

There are two kinds of surgical ear procedures: otoplasty, or ear pinning, which is done for overly large ears whose cartilage sticks out, and earlobe reduction. Both of these procedures are permanent.

Otoplasty is a quick procedure, usually taking one hour, and is performed under local anesthesia for most of my adult patients. During otoplasty, an incision is made just behind the ear in the natural fold where it joins with the head. After the skin is lifted off the cartilage, it is reshaped using stitches to hold it permanently in place. This surgery can be done after the ears reach 80 percent of their full size, around the age of five or six. In fact, this is one procedure in which the earlier it's done, the better (Figure 63).

Earlobe reduction surgery is also a quick procedure, typically taking thirty minutes. The surgery is performed using either the wedge reduction method or the peripheral margin

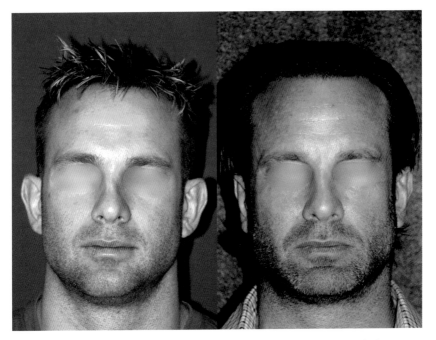

Figure 63: Before (left) and after (right) of a man who underwent an otoplasty, or ear pinning procedure. The altered ears frame the face better, as prominent ears can distract from other facial features.

reduction method. I do not recommend the wedge reduction method, because taking a wedge out of the earlobe will make it look smaller but also narrower, and a narrow earlobe looks awkward. The peripheral margin reduction allows the doctor to control shape and size. I hand my patients a mirror and tell them to show me what size and shape they want their earlobes to be, and we draw this on the earlobe itself. The extra gets removed by following the drawn-on pattern, and the edges are sutured together. The incision is on the edge of the newly created earlobe so the scars cannot be seen (Figure 64).

If there has been a lot of damage to the earlobe from earrings, it is common to reduce the earlobe and to close stretched-out earring holes by trimming the skin in the tract of the earring hole and suturing it together. The earlobes then cannot be re-pierced for six weeks.

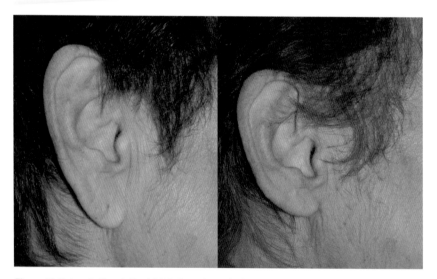

Figure 64: Before (left) and after (right) of a patient who had earlobe reduction surgery. As we age, the earlobes become longer and more pendulous. The earlobe size and shape can be customized in this procedure.

What to Expect After Ear Surgery

Ear procedures typically result in minimal bruising and swelling. Most of my patients can go back to work the next day. If you've had an otoplasty and have short, ear-revealing hair, know that bruising can last up to five days, so you may want to take a few more days off work.

Restoring Your Hairline

Hair loss can be devastating, for men and for women. There's no way to hide it, unless you get a wig or extensions—and extensions can actually accelerate hair loss, as their weight damages the healthy hair follicles you still have. For a long time, hair plugs were the only option. It's a terrible process, requiring groups of twenty or more hairs to be removed at a time, and placed back into the scalp in a way that looks wholly unnatural. It is painful and tedious, and it leaves scars. Hair plugs have left many people thinking that hair transplants are all about secretly leaving the surgeon's office with their heads wrapped in bandages, then going home to heal with significant bleeding and discomfort. All of this was endured to end up with a scalp that looks like it was studded with rooted doll hair.

Fortunately, hair replacement for men and women has gone high-tech and is now much easier to do than in the old days of hair plugs—with much more natural results.

What Happens to Your Hair as You Age

As we age, the rate of hair growth slows. Both men and women suffer hair loss, but patterns may differ between them. The most common cause of thinning hair is heredity, passed down from either your mother's or your father's side of the family. You may notice areas of hair that no longer need cutting, where the hairs are getting shorter and finer. It is important to know that finding hairs in your tub, sink, or brush is not necessarily a sign of thinning hair; they could indicate a temporary hair loss condition. It is natural for hair to go through a constant cycle of growth and resting, or dormancy. If you are not on your way to balding, your hair will grow back just as strong. If you are balding, your hair will grow back finer, not growing as long before falling out again. What you see in the mirror over a longer period is the best monitor of early signs of thinning.

MALE PATTERN BALDNESS

It is estimated that 50 million men in the United States are affected by male pattern baldness, or androgenetic alopecia.[2] "Andro" refers to the androgen hormones (testosterone and dihydrotestosterone, or DHT) necessary to produce male pattern hair loss; "genetic" refers to the inherited gene necessary for male pattern hair loss to occur. In men who develop male pattern baldness, hair loss may begin any time after puberty, when androgen levels increase. The first change is usually recession around the temples, which is seen in 96 percent of mature Caucasian males, including those men lucky enough not to progress to further hair loss.[3] Later, the frontal hairline recedes, resulting ultimately in a classic horseshoe-shaped fringe of hair and a bald crown and frontal hairline. Whether this happens in the twenties, thirties, forties, fifties, or beyond is related to genetic factors, and inheritance can be from one's mother, father, or even grandparent.

FEMALE PATTERN BALDNESS

In female pattern balding, the hair thins all over the head, but the frontal hairline is maintained. There may be a moderate loss of hair on the crown, but this rarely progresses to near or total baldness. Female pattern balding is primarily genetic in origin but can be caused by hormonal changes or abnormalities, certain diseases, and various medical and dietary interventions. If you notice you are losing a lot of hair, it's time to see your physician or an endocrinologist to rule out any underlying medical condition. If there are no other causes of hair loss diagnosed, a surgical hair transplant is an excellent option.

Nonsurgical Hair Restoration Procedures

There are many products for sale that promise nonsurgical hair restoration. At some point in our lives we all will experience at least some mild thinning of the hair, so hair restoration is a big business. In fact, there are very few nonsurgical treatments that have been shown to be effective. I want to shed light on these treatments so that you can save your money and ignore products that promise a lot but can't deliver.

There are only three at-home treatments that I have identified that work at all: Nutrafol, Rogaine, and Propecia. Nutrafol is a dietary product that is designed to nourish and strengthen thinning hair from within. It is formulated with botanical ingredients that are clinically proven. It features the latest technology that standardizes the ingredients to specifically target the multiple triggers of hair loss. Hair loss has various causes, including inflammation, hormones, stress, and genetics. Therefore, to address the problem, a sophisticated, multi-targeting formula is required, and Nutrafol fits this bill.

It begins by balancing the level of DHT and cortisol hormones, then repairs damaged follicles, ultimately revitalizing dormant follicles by providing them with nutrients and building blocks necessary to promote hair growth. This results in healthy, fuller, stronger hair. There are two different formulations for men and for women. Here are some of the ingredients used in the formula and their benefits:

Hydrolyzed fish collagen rebuilds your follicle environment, improves moisture, and promotes diffusion of nutrients.

Ashwagandha, the plant *Withania somnifera* (also known as Indian ginseng), decreases the level of cortisol stress hormones.

Hyaluronic acid helps to keep your hair moisturized throughout.

Bioperine aids in the optimal absorption of potent ingredients.

Biotin strengthens your hair as well as improves its overall health.

Saw palmetto reduces the action of the enzyme responsible for hair loss.

Amino acid blend provides you with building blocks for healthy and strong hair.

Nutrafol can be purchased online and is sold in dermatologists' and plastic surgeons' offices across the country. While it is not a cure-all, it is a complete formulation that ensures you do not have any nutritional deficiencies that may enable hair loss. I strongly suggest it to all my patients worried about hair loss. It is reasonably priced at $88 a month.

Minoxidil, or Rogaine, is one of the only FDA-approved topical treatments for hair loss that is available over the counter. Minoxidil does stimulate hair growth, but not the coarse hair that we want. It stimulates what is called vellus hair, which is similar to the fine hair on the back of your neck. I have spoken to thousands of patients using minoxidil who have not experienced significant growth of the hair that matters. I would tell you that it cannot hurt, and it may possibly prevent further hair loss, but you will likely need to do something else if you are looking to regrow or thicken your head of hair.

Propecia (or finasteride) is an oral medication that is commonly prescribed for hair loss. It inhibits an enzyme that converts testosterone to a form that will trigger male pattern hair loss. I prescribed this medication for years, because it can affect hair regrowth and prevent further hair loss with long-term use. I stopped prescribing the drug when a study out of Northwestern University showed that finasteride can cause long-term sexual dysfunction, persisting even after users have stopped taking the drug.[4] It is my opinion that this is too great a price to pay, especially because the side effects can be irreversible.

There are several light stimulation devices for hair regrowth that are sold for thousands of dollars. These include laser combs, laser hats, and LED devices, none of which have shown any efficacy in randomized controlled trials. Although it seems like lasers are cure-all devices, in this case they are not. I would avoid these and spend your money elsewhere.

Another minimally invasive treatment that shows promise for hair loss is platelet-rich plasma, also known as PRP. It uses a solution created with a high concentration of platelets, which are administered to the scalp via an injection. These injections of PRP are used to stimulate and promote healthy tissue regeneration. The platelets used in the PRP treatments are naturally found in the human body and work by repairing damaged tissue. They also stimulate the body's own stem cells to move toward the tissue damage to help in the repair process.

PRP is created by drawing your blood, which is then run through a centrifuge machine. The centrifuge machine spins the blood around at a high speed, which in turn separates out the red and white blood cells from the platelets. The result is a high concentration of platelet-rich plasma, which contains three to five times the normal number of platelets found in blood. It also contains PDGF (platelet-derived growth factor), VEGF (vascular endothelial growth factor), TGF (transforming growth factor), and other proteins that help with soft tissue healing. To activate the PRP after it is injected in the scalp, we will stimulate the hair follicles by microneedling the scalp. I usually suggest three treatment sessions separated by six weeks each (Figure 65).

Patients generally see new hair growth within four to six months following their PRP injections, with hair continuing

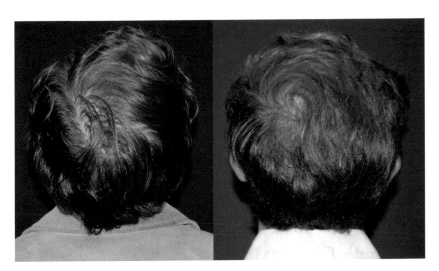

Figure 65: Before (left) and after (right) of a patient who had platelet-rich plasma (PRP) injections to the scalp to regrow thinning hair. The PRP is derived from your blood and multiple treatments are required.

to thicken over the following year. Thicker and denser hair is typically noticeable in the treated area and especially evident in the hairline. Results last up to a year and can be prolonged with follow-up PRP treatments.

I suggest these treatments for those who are just starting to lose hair as more of a preventative treatment. For patients with more advanced balding, I have found PRP to be less effective, with significant results visible in only 50 percent of treatments.

Surgical Hair Restoration Procedures

For All Ethnicities

Choosing hair restoration surgery is a major decision for most people and will permanently change their appearances for the better. Older technology used "plugs" with groups of twenty or more hairs, which made hair transplantation very obvious, almost making the hair appear like "doll's hair" coming out of the scalp of a child's toy. Now, hair transplant surgery is so advanced that the restored hair will actually grow naturally. You can get it cut and styled like the hair you used to have. Your hairline will look and function as if it is untouched. It really is that undetectable.

The essence of these procedures is that the hair is transplanted into the balding area as individual follicular units. If you look closely under magnification, you can see that hair grows in clusters of one, two, three, and sometimes four hairs. These naturally occurring groups of hair are called follicular hair units. We can transfer these follicles to be placed closer together to create a denser-looking head of hair. Micrografting is a delicate and time-consuming process. Each follicular hair unit has to be kept intact and trimmed under a microscope to create the ultimate micro graft. The end result is a hair transplant that can be undetectable. Follicular unit grafts require more time and skill, and a dedicated, well-trained staff, compared to the mini grafts that were traditionally performed. This technique may entail five assistants working with microscopes for many hours or even the whole day. Once transplanted, the hairs continue to grow for a lifetime.

There are two ways to harvest the hair from the back of the scalp: the strip method and follicular unit extraction (Figure 66). With the strip method, a section of scalp is surgically removed and the area is stitched up, creating a linear scar on the back of the head that fades over time. The strip of scalp is

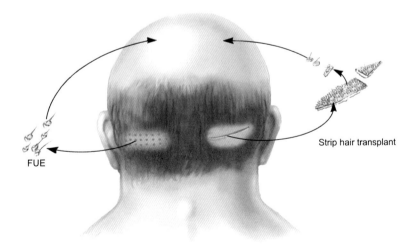

Figure 66: There are two types of hair transplant methods. The strip procedure surgically removes a piece of your scalp, leaving a linear scar. Follicular unit extraction (FUE) removes each hair follicle individually so that there is minimal visible scarring. Many patients today opt for FUE.

then dissected under the microscope, removing each individual hair follicle. This is a better option when it's not practical for you to have an area of your head shaved, which is required in the follicular unit extraction method. In strip surgery, the hair from above and below the incision covers the area so that it is not visible immediately after the procedure. Patients often go back to work the day after surgery. This technique is more painful, however, due to the incision line. It is ideal for men who do not shave their heads or wear super-short haircuts. In short and bald hairstyles, the incisions from the strip procedure will be visible because they do not completely disappear.

In follicular unit extraction (FUE), a relatively large area in the back and sides of the scalp is shaved to approximately 1 millimeter in length. Instead of removing a single strip, a tiny circular incision is made, using a fine needle–sized instrument, around each follicular unit in order to extract it. I use a NeoGraft device for this. One advantage of the NeoGraft system is that it is virtually painless. There is no scalpel, no cutting, no staples, and no scarring. The hair takes root right away. The tiny wounds are left open to heal on their own, not requiring any stitches to close. They heal with no linear or appreciable scarring so you could shave your head and nobody would know you had a hair transplant.

If you've lost a lot of hair, you may need multiple sessions. The maximum number of hair grafts you can do in a day is 2,500 to 3,000, which is called a mega-session. This takes an entire day because it is a slow and delicate process, literally splitting the hairs. Depending on the degree of balding, and the degree of hair density desired, patients may require up to two or three mega-sessions. In female pattern baldness, the goal is to create more hair density over large areas of the scalp so multiple mega-sessions are certainly required. For men, the first few transplant sessions are usually done in the front of the hairline above the forehead, to frame the face. The subsequent sessions focus on the crown. Those who are only balding in the crown can have just that area treated.

Whether you harvest the hair as a strip or with NeoGraft, the recipient sites are made, and the follicular unit grafts are carefully inserted into the scalp. The one-hair grafts are placed at the hairline, the two-hairs immediately behind them, and the larger three- and four-hair units are placed in the central forelock area. The artistry in hair transplantation is in how

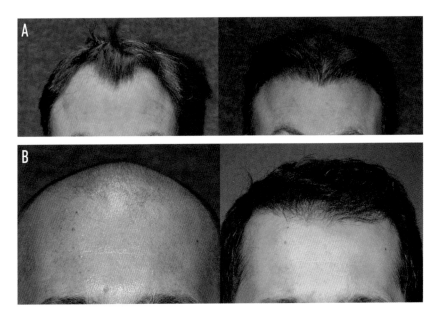

Figure 67: Before (left) and after (right) of hair transplant. Frontal hairline replacement with a natural nongeometric pattern.

the surgeon blends and shapes the hairline. If the hairline is constructed like a straight edge, it will appear artificial. The hairline needs to have a natural wave, mimicking your original hairline, and should not be placed too low (Figure 67).

What to Expect After Hair Restoration Surgery

Most hair restoration procedures are performed under local anesthesia, which means no general anesthesia and therefore a quick recovery that will not affect your ability to go back to work. Hair transplant sessions that use thousands of follicular unit grafts may take a whole day; however, the time goes by quickly. During the procedure, patients rest comfortably and can watch TV or a movie, take a nap, or chat with the staff.

The misperceptions that people may have of hair transplantation, in which patients leave the office with their heads wrapped in bandages and with significant bleeding and pain, derive from experience with outdated plug techniques. In modern follicular unit hair transplants, patients leave the office with only a hat and headband.

While facial structure and hair procedures may seem overwhelming, I hope this chapter puts some myths and misperceptions to rest. Advancements in technology have radically changed the way we approach some of these procedures, while others may sound familiar to you by now. As always, the key to safe and effective treatments is simple: preparation. If you know what to expect and you trust your skilled and

experienced surgeon, you'll leave the office after your procedure feeling even more confident than when you entered.

1 Darrick Antell, "How CEOs Lead with Their Chins," *BusinessWeek* via Antell MD (2008), https://
www.antell-md.com/businesswk08.html.

2 "Androgenetic alopecia," Genetics Home Reference, 2018, https://ghr.nlm.nih.gov/condition/
androgenetic-alopecia#statistics.

3 Karyn Springer et al., "Common Hair Loss Disorders," *American Family Physician* 68, no. 1
(2003), 93–102, https://www.aafp.org/afp/2003/0701/p93.html.

4 Tina Kiguradze et al., "Persistent Erectile Dysfunction in Men Exposed to the 5α-reductase
Inhibitors, Finasteride, or Dutasteride," *PeerJ* 5 (2017), e3020, doi: 10.7717/peerj.3020, https://
www.ncbi.nlm.nih.gov/pubmed/28289563.

10 Jawlines and Necks That Defy Gravity

For many of my patients, one of the most dreaded, telltale signs of aging is the "turkey neck." The late Nora Ephron even wrote a book entitled *I Feel Bad About My Neck*—a title millions of people can identify with. Many of my patients tell me that when they look in the mirror, all they can see is the extra loose skin of their necks, the vertical bands in the center of their necks, and the jowls beginning to develop where there once was a crisp jawline. Fortunately, there are many options to fix this and make you feel good about your jawline and neck again. This chapter will discuss the best nonsurgical and surgical treatments to smooth and tighten your jawline and neck.

What Happens to Your Jawline and Neck as You Age

As we age, the constant pull of gravity creates more skin that hangs, excess fat begins to deposit deep under the skin below the chin, and the facial and neck muscles loosen. As you've probably noticed already, diet and exercise can do little to improve the difficult area below the chin. This fat grows due to hormonal changes that occur with aging and has nothing to do with weight.

These changes most commonly produce the following effects:

- double chin
- loose, sagging jowls
- sagging neck skin, or "turkey wattle"
- hanging neck muscles that appear like ropey vertical bands
- crêpe-like texture in the neck skin

The skin on the neck is not quite the same as facial skin, as there are fewer oil-producing skin cells (which is why it's rare to develop acne on your neck). With less moisturizing from the skin itself, its texture is compromised, becoming dry and crêpey.

The platysma is a broad sheet of muscles positioned on each side of the neck. It is divided into two separate and distinct sides, with the right and left platysma muscle meeting in the center of the neck. As we age, the tissue and fibers that connect the platysma to the overlying skin begin to weaken and lose their elasticity. The connection between the two platysma muscles also weakens and separates as the muscles sag. As a result, you usually begin to see two vertical muscle bands in the neck starting in your late forties and early fifties, which worsen with age. These neck muscles are continuous with a muscle in the lower third of the face called the superficial musculo aponeurotic system (SMAS).

There are both nonsurgical and surgical ways to treat these layers, which I will describe in this chapter, revealing the true efficacy and limitations of each. There are also many devices on the market producing results that are subtle and modest at best. It is important to know what you are purchasing because these treatments can be very costly, and if they do not deliver adequate outcomes, it's highly likely that you will wind up spending more money on a treatment that does.

Nonsurgical Jawline and Neck Procedures

All nonsurgical devices that tighten the lower third of the face, jawline, and neck work using the same principle: They deliver thermal (heat) energy to the layers of the face and neck (i.e., the skin, muscle, and fat), causing them to contract and tighten. This thermal energy also stimulates collagen production in the deep layers of the skin (the dermis) while leaving the skin's surface (the epidermis) relatively untouched. The best analogy to help describe this is when we throw a pair of pants in the dryer and the heat makes the fabric shrink so they fit more snugly. Similarly, the heat energy delivered by these devices will make our loosening face and neck tissues tighten along the jawline. There are two main sources of energy used to impart this thermal effect: radiofrequency and ultrasound (Figure 68). What follows is a dissection of the newest devices that deliver this energy, some without penetrating the skin surface at all and others in a minimally invasive way.

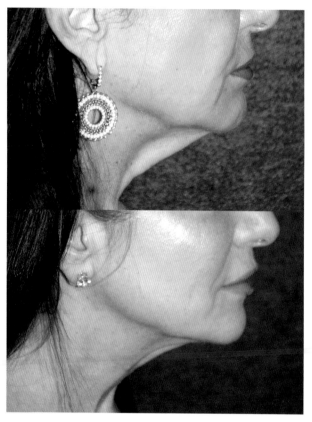

Figure 68: Before (top) and after (bottom) of nonsurgical neck tightening using deep tissue heating. These results can be accomplished with Ulthera, ThermiTight, and FaceTite.

LOOSE SKIN AND MUSCLES

RADIOFREQUENCY ENERGY

Radiofrequency (RF) waves are used to deliver thermal (heat) energy to the face. The first set of external RF devices discussed below use a probe that sits on the surface of the skin. Radiofrequency devices are either monopolar (with one pole on the probe delivering the radiofrequency waves) or bipolar (with two poles), the most common being Thermage, Titan, and Aluma.

I have owned Thermage and Titan machines, and my experience with external radiofrequency skin tightening is that the results are not very predictable. The results are usually extremely subtle, but there are a significant number of people whom I have treated who had no visible result at all. Most RF results are not visible right away, taking place gradually, over a period of several weeks or months as the new collagen forms.

Today there are more effective internal RF devices that use a probe that penetrates the skin, thus delivering the thermal energy to the deeper layers of the tissues. Although not technically surgery with incisions and sutures, it is a minimally invasive procedure where the probe is moved back and forth under the skin through a small hole in the skin. The three main types of internal RF are microneedling RF, ThermiTight, and FaceTite.

With microneedling RF, the probe has small pins (microneedles) that enter the skin imparting radiofrequency. So, you're getting both the physical injury, as you do with all microneedling devices, and also the added heat effect. The heat creates thermal zones beyond the actual reach of the needle. While this is more effective than a surface probe, resulting in better skin tightening, it still has limited effects on the underlying fat and muscles.

ThermiTight uses a small electrode inserted under the skin to heat tissue to a clinician-selected therapeutic temperature. After a small volume of anesthetic solution is injected into the area to be treated, the tiny ThermiTight SmartTip thermistor probe is inserted under the skin. The surgeon applies gentle movements to heat up the tissues to the desired level. Skin safety is monitored with Thermal Image Guidance. Most procedures last less than one hour. Because the thermal energy is delivered with the probe under the skin within the subcutaneous (under the skin) fat layer, it melts away excess fat in all areas of your lower face, jawline, and neck. It is not surgery, but some mild bruising does occur. The probe also glides over the surface of the muscles, thermally tightening them as well, which is why it can be much more effective than the older generation of RF devices (whose probes simply sit on the surface of the skin).

Another RF device, having recently arrived on the market, is FaceTite. It combines internal delivery of RF energy, with a probe placed under the skin (like ThermiTight), and another external probe placed on the surface of the skin (like Thermage). The deep tissues and the skin surface are treated at the same time, with a sandwich of heating. Theoretically, the dual-attack treatment should result in better tightening than other RF technologies, but this has not been shown in clinical studies. However, FaceTite does provide unprecedented skin contraction, with up to 36 percent shown in peer-reviewed clinical studies. Perhaps because of this, patient satisfaction is high and the outcomes are probably the best in the nonsurgical neck lift category.

One thing to keep in mind regarding radiofrequency tightening is that if you have more significant, heavy jowls, due to genetics or advancing age, the results are more limited and you may not be a good candidate. As we get older, our faces become like a baggy pair of pants. If they are one size too big

ThermiTight Quick Facts

ThermiTight may be the perfect touch-up procedure for patients who have already had a facelift. Here are five facts about ThermiTight to consider when choosing the RF treatment right for you:

- results can appear instantly and continue to improve over six to twelve months, ultimately lasting from three to five years
- more affordable than a full facelift
- performed right in the office, with no surgical suite needed
- causes minimal scarring and bruising
- requires short downtime, with most patients returning to work the next day

and you put them in the dryer, they will shrink enough to fit well. This is like a patient in their forties to early fifties whose face is just a little lax. But if the pair of jeans is three sizes too big, the heat of the dryer will not tighten them up enough and the pants will still be baggy. This is like a patient who has a turkey neck and jowls, for whom these noninvasive treatments will leave the face too "baggy" or "droopy."

ULTRASONIC ENERGY

Another form of energy used to tighten the neck skin is ultrasound. Ulthera is the first and only ultrasound energy–based device cleared by the FDA with a noninvasive "lift" indication for the neck, face, and eyebrows. Ultrasound is sound at frequencies higher than those detected by human hearing (at least 18 kilohertz or 18,000 cycles per second). Ultherapy addresses the deep skin layers as well as the foundational layer that lends support to the skin. This foundational layer in the face is called the SMAS, and, in the neck, the platysma. Ultrasound allows me to bypass the upper layers of the skin and deliver the right amount of energy at the right depths to contract and then ultimately lift the SMAS and platysma. The main advantage of Ultherapy over ThermiTight and FaceTite is that you do not have to put the probe under the skin to treat the fat and muscle layer. As a result, there is no damage on the surface of the skin and thus no healing downtime. This treatment takes approximately one hour. However, it can be painful, so my patients are given ibuprofen or another painkiller before treatment to minimize discomfort.

The full effect of Ultherapy will build gradually over the course of two to three months. After the first month, you may experience slight lifting and toning, a tighter, firmer feel, and a smoother texture. Over the next two to three months, you may experience tighter skin with reduced sagging, a sleeker jawline, and improved contour under the chin.

Ultherapy works best for those who are beginning to show signs of skin laxity and jowls, especially around the jawline. How well it works depends on different factors, including how lax your skin already is, its volume (or fat distribution), its texture (extent of lines, wrinkles, crêpiness, and/or sun damage),

Thread Lifts: Full Disclosure

One procedure I do not recommend is the thread lift. Thread lifts have been around for more than fifteen years and were originally distributed by a company that sold a product called Contour Threads. The threads were made of a permanent suture material (prolene), studded with little barbs to catch facial skin and tissue. Contour Threads were inserted under the skin through a small incision, into the droopy areas of the jawline and neck, then pulled up and secured to a stable muscle in front of the ear for the jowls, and behind the ear for the neck. The company discontinued the product because of patient dissatisfaction; the results did not last long and patients could feel the permanent threads through the skin. I was an early adopter of this procedure because so many of my patients wanted to try it, but I stopped performing thread lifts one year after I started. I found that the results were only lasting nine months, and the procedure was costly to patients.

In the last few years, another company has introduced a new type of thread lift, called the Silhouette InstaLift. It is an FDA-cleared technology, and the company claims that it provides an immediate facelift effect as well as a regenerative effect for progressive and natural results. Silhouette InstaLift works by placing a biodegradable thread with absorbable cones (instead of barbs) into the subcutaneous fat layer just beneath the skin where the lifting is desired. Like Contour Threads, Silhouette thread is placed under your skin, catching the droopy skin, and is then lifted up and secured. The company claims that the results last at least eighteen months, with many patients reporting more than two years of effectiveness. Even though I do not perform thread lifts anymore, I doubt that the results with these threads last longer than the six to nine months the old version produced. In fact, it stands to reason that the new treatments last for even less time, because the threads reabsorb over a few months. I have attended lectures by plastic surgery colleagues of mine who have performed hundreds of these Silhouette Lifts, and, to be completely blunt, the results are so subtle that sometimes I cannot tell the difference between the before-and-after photos they show.

In short, I would not suggest a thread lift unless you have a specific event you'd like to prepare for, such as your child's wedding, and you do not want surgery. In this case, I'd recommend procuring the procedure six to eight weeks before the event, but don't expect results to last more than a few months.

your age, and your lifestyle and health (i.e., smoking habits, nature of health issues). Improvements range from a 10 to 20 percent tightening. Patients with thin skin, a defined jawline, strong cheek and chin structure, and less facial fat tend to have the best results, while those with a rounded or heavy face, thick skin, and weak skeletal structure show less improvement.

DOUBLE CHINS AND NECK FAT

There are currently two available methods of nonsurgically reducing neck fat: injections with Kybella and CoolSculpting.

KYBELLA

Kybella, as described in Chapter 5, consists of bile acids that literally digest the fat under your neck. It was created to treat excessive fullness and localized fatty tissue underneath the chin, and it's an excellent example of how marketing can create buzz around a device or procedure whose results can't live up to the hype. The regimen requires up to five monthly treatments of multiple injections—as many as fifty of them per session. What Kybella's very clever marketing campaign fails to mention is that, after the material is injected, your neck blows up like a bullfrog for three to five days. So, it is not wash-and-wear; there is a significant recovery time. In fact, if you do it three times, we're talking a total of fifteen days of recovery.

Kybella works best on patients in their thirties and forties whose skin still has a lot of elasticity and easily snaps back. The results are also permanent, as once the fat cells break down, they can't ever re-form. The problem I have found with Kybella is that the results are often disappointing for those with lax or drooping skin. When the fat is dissolved, the skin will still hang (think about the hanging, excessive belly skin left after massive weight loss). If you have a lot of redundant skin under your chin, without good elasticity, Kybella can make it hang even *more*.

COOLSCULPTING

CoolSculpting has been used in more than two million neck and body treatments worldwide to date. CoolSculpting works by a process called cryolipolysis, in which freezing fat cells causes them to die; it's like frostbite for fat. To achieve a 20 percent reduction in under-chin fat, a patient must submit to one or two sixty-minute sessions. During the session, the neck fat is clamped into the curved jaws of the CoolMini probe of the machine. The arctic-level cold quickly numbs the area, making pain during treatment negligible, but there can be post-treatment pain, swelling, redness, and bruising. (Nerve pain that persisted for several weeks has been reported anecdotally by patients following CoolSculpting of the abdomen.)

FDA clearance of the CoolMini was based on a trial involving sixty male and female patients, ages twenty-two to sixty-five. In a press release, the company stated that "no significant adverse events were observed and patients experienced little or no discomfort or downtime." Patients in the study saw results at three weeks, but the best results were observed after one to three months. The problems with CoolSculpting are the same as those with Kybella. You only get a partial correction of the neck fat (20 percent), requiring multiple treatments, which become very expensive. CoolScupting also results in the same loose skin issue for patients in their late forties and older.

When it comes to removing stubborn neck fat, neck liposuction is more efficient and likely less costly than Kybella or CoolSculpting, as you'll see in the next section.

Surgical Jawline and Neck Procedures

For All Ethnicities

There are several different kinds of surgery that treat jawline and neck issues. There are three components to what makes the neck look heavy: extra fat under the chin, which can be removed with liposuction; vertical banding of the muscle bands, or platysmal, in the neck, which can be treated with a corset platysmaplasty; and loose skin, which can be removed with a neck lift. There are two different neck lift procedures that can be performed: an isolated neck lift and a direct neck lift. A more complete facelift, as you'll see in the next chapter, will lift the jowls completely, whereas the surgical procedures we are focusing on in this chapter specifically target the jawline and neck.

Submental or neck liposuction removes excess fatty tissue to help further define the chin and the neckline, often referred to as double chin surgery. When the skin heals, the muscles of the neck contract and tighten up, meaning the neck contour will improve by both volume reduction and tissue tightening. To remove the fat, a tiny incision is made beneath the chin and behind each ear. Using a small device called a cannula, the fat is suctioned away. It is important to perform the liposuction from three approaches; if you go in only from the midline under the chin, you will not get as defined a contour along the whole jawline, including where the jawbone starts, by your ear. I perform submental liposuction under local anesthesia, with numbing shots like the Novocain you get at the dentist.

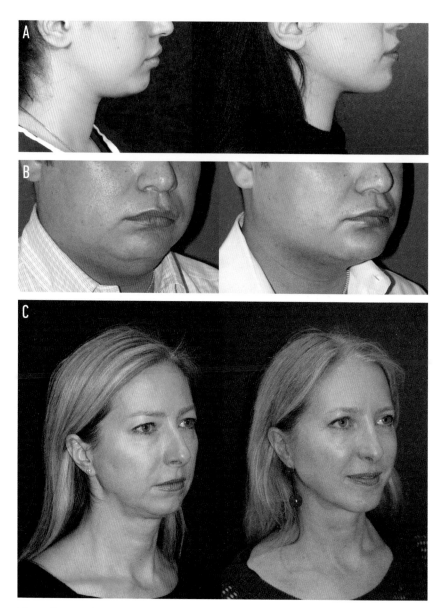

Figure 69: Before (left) and after (right) of patients after submental (neck) liposuction. A) Female patient. B) Male patient. C) Aging female patient who also had a concomitant upper and lower eyelid lift and chin implant. Liposuction can be helpful as the neck skin loosens, but if there is too much skin it can sag after you reduce the fat so that a neck lift may be necessary as you get older.

The recovery generally lasts about five days and the treatment is complete in one session (Figure 69). The recovery from non-invasive fat reduction procedures is about the same, and you have to do them multiple times. For this reason, I think doing liposuction is a more efficient and better value than Kybella or CoolSculpting.

If there is more advanced loosening of the platysma muscle in the neck, creating vertical bands and cords, liposuction will not do enough to result in a beautiful neck contour. In this case, a corset platysmaplasty neck lift is performed in combination with the liposuction. First, neck liposuction is completed. The platysmaplasty neck lift is then performed by making a 1-centimeter (or 3/8 of an inch) incision discreetly hidden under your chin. Through this small incision, a fiber optic telescope called an endoscope is used to visualize and operate on the deeper fat planes and loosening muscles that have developed (Figure 70). The excess fat that cannot be accessed with lipo-suction, called the inter-platysmal and sub-platysmal fat, is reduced; excess, loose platysma muscle is removed; and the left and right platysma muscles are reconnected in the center of the neck (like a corset undergarment). By joining them together, the muscle that was sagging tightens up under the chin, creat-ing a single sheet of muscle, called a midline platysma plica-tion. This tightened single sheet of platysma muscle will flatten the neck bands. Those patients with moderate aging of the neck (usually between the ages of forty and the late fifties) are the best candidates for a platysmaplasty. Recovery and bruis-ing last five to seven days and can be covered by wearing a

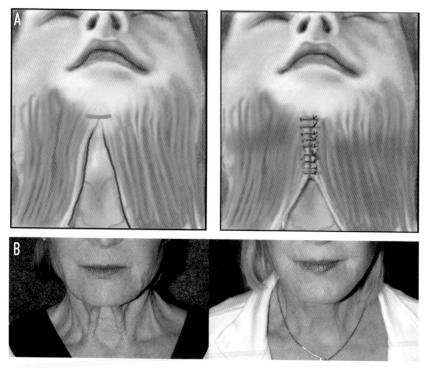

Figure 70: A) Incision for a platysmaplasty and demonstration of tightening vertical bands of muscle in the neck. B) Before (left) and after (right) of a patient who had a platysmaplasty.

collared shirt or a scarf around the neck. Similar to neck liposuction, the platysmaplasty procedure does not remove excess skin. With more significant aging and a heavier drooping neck, the platysmaplasty must be combined with a neck lift surgery that will further tighten the platysma and remove drooping, excess neck skin.

We have spent most of the chapter describing either nonsurgical or less invasive surgical procedures that partially correct or improve the neck in an attempt to avoid a neck lift, which is perceived as a more major surgery. The truth is, the recovery time for a neck lift is similar to that of a neck liposuction or corset platyamplasty. Neck lifts do not require general anesthesia and are performed by making an incision behind the ears, so no scars are visible. The operative time is twice as long, about an hour to an hour and a half, because the approach behind each ear is combined with the corset platysmaplasty procedure described above. Through the incision behind each ear, the outer part of the platysma muscle is lifted and secured, sliding it backward into its original youthful position (Figure 71). Thus, the muscle is tightened on the sides of the neck and also in the middle of the neck. This technique results in less bruising and swelling since it lifts beneath the muscle and not the skin where all the bruising occurs. Once the deeper tissue is lifted, the excess skin is trimmed and re-sutured. Scars

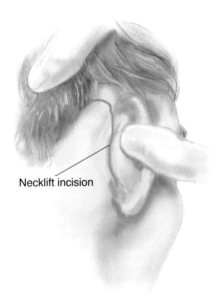

Necklift incision

Figure 71: Incisions for a neck lift are hidden behind the ears. The extra hanging neck skin is removed here and the neck platysma muscle tightened.

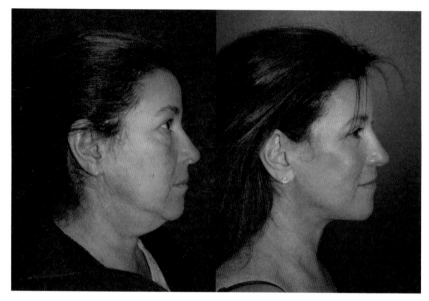

Figure 72: Before (left) and after (right) of a female patient who underwent a neck lift. She had an upper and lower eyelid lift performed at the same time.

heal better because there is no tension on superficial layers and skin. This lift results in a natural, softer look and creates definition along the jawline and neck (Figure 72).

JAWLINE AND NECK PROCEDURES FOR MEN

As men get older, especially those in the business world who need to wear a suit and tie every day to work, they often find their necks drooping at their collars. Men are as sensitive about their turkey necks as women are, but, in my experience, they usually don't want a neck lift as described above. Instead, for these patients, I perform a direct neck lift, in which the skin is removed directly under the chin in the middle of the neck and not behind the ears. Because men have bearded skin, the incision on the neck heals well and is camouflaged, but the

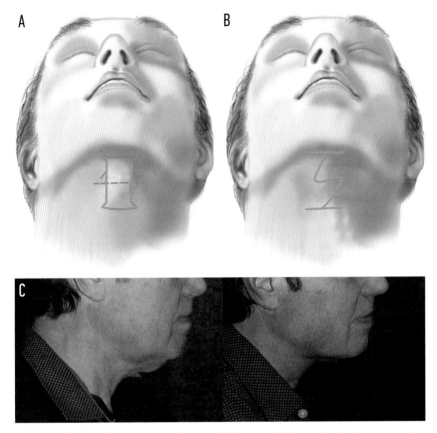

Figure 73: A) Incision for a Grecian urn direct neck lift for men. B) Closure of neck skin removal with z-plasty. C) Before (left) and after (right) of a male patient who had a Grecian urn direct neck lift. The recovery for this is quicker than for a traditional neck lift. The bearded skin of the male neck camouflages the incisions well.

scars would be unsightly on women. The skin is excised in a complex pattern that removes both vertical and horizontal skin excess in a pattern called a "Grecian urn," and incorporates a z-plasty (creating a Z in the incision) to camouflage the scar (Figure 73). This skin removal provides access to the deep neck fat and allows me to tighten the sagging platysma with a corset platysmaplasty. The immediate effect is that the jawline looks more defined, and most people will comment that you look like you have lost weight because the heaviness under the neck has been removed.

I have done this surgery on hundreds of men who can't take a lot of time off work. This is a good option, as it only needs a four- to five-day recuperation, with a few bandages placed over the incision. If anyone asks what happened, it's easy enough to say a cyst was removed if the patient prefers not to discuss having had surgery.

BOTCHED NECK SURGERY: WHAT CAN GO WRONG AND HOW TO FIX IT

Liposuction only works in patients without a lot of extra skin or with skin that still has a lot of elasticity. If the skin is excessive, it will end up hanging loosely and the patient will be very unhappy. If the muscles under the neck are loose and not addressed with a platysmaplasty, removing the fat that hides the platysma banding will actually make them more visible.

I have seen many overdone neck lifts with dramatic results that are the opposite of what the surgery intended. The necklines look carved out and not soft, making them appear manipulated and sculpted, as opposed to youthful. This mistake can occur when a surgeon performs overly aggressive liposuction, where all of the fat is removed from the neck. The skin then heals down to the muscle layer so the skin looks tucked in. None of the softening characteristics of a small, thin blanket of fat under the skin are present, which can be avoided by using a smaller liposuction cannula. This unwanted result is very difficult to reverse, but it can be attempted by injecting fat harvested from the body (abdomen, flanks, or thighs) under the skin in layers. The fat usually only partially takes in this area, so two or more fat transfer sessions are required.

Another excessive neck lift attribute is neck skin that appears taut and stretched, not smooth. This happens when the neck skin is lifted and removed behind the ears without lifting the platysma muscle on the sides of the neck. Many plastic surgeons who do not specialize in facial surgery are not comfortable with lifting the platysma muscle (because of their fear of blood vessels, nerves, and deeper structures) and make this mistake. Since the muscle is not lifted, all the tension of the neck lift repair is on the skin and not on the muscle, creating a cadaver-like look that is not rejuvenating even though no neck skin is hanging. The only way to repair this is to repeat the incision behind the ears, lifting the muscle to take the tension off the skin.

The last and most difficult problem to correct is something called the "cobra neck deformity." This happens when too much of the deep fat is removed under the platysma, and the platysma muscles of the central neck are also excessively removed. The result is a neck that appears like the head of a cobra, with the center of the neck gauged out and two hanging platysma muscles on the left and right sides (Figure 74). Correcting this requires a complex repair, where muscles deep to the platysma muscles, called the digastrics, are mobilized and sutured in to the depth of the hole in the center of the neck, and the residual platysma muscle is moved to the center of the

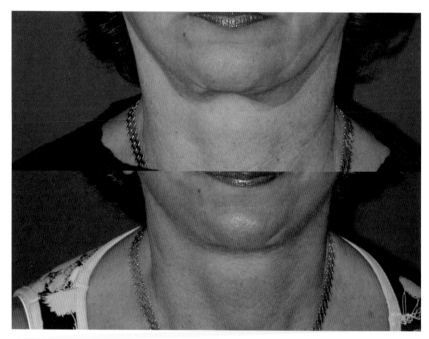

Figure 74: Before (top) and after (bottom) of corrective surgery for a cobra neck deformity that occurs from too much tissue removal during a neck lift (performed elsewhere). To repair this, the platysma muscle of the neck needs to be used to fill the void.

neck and sutured to each other (as in a corset platysmaplasty). It differs from a typical corset procedure because the platysma muscle repair must be stabilized, requiring suturing to the central hyoid bone in the middle of the neck. Recovery is longer from this procedure, so, to say the least, it is best to avoid this complication.

What to Expect After Jawline and Neck Surgery

Immediately after surgery, patients may experience a tight feeling in the neck, which is extremely normal and will subside gradually as the healing process continues over three to four weeks. The neck skin will feel numb for a few months as well. You *should* avoid heavy lifting or strenuous activities for two weeks to ensure the best possible results.

While one of the procedures described in this chapter might be the perfect choice for you, it remains true that all of them are viewed as alternatives to a traditional facelift. Depending on your body and your needs, these jawline and neck treatments can be extremely effective, and I regularly recommend and perform them. However, if you know you're a good candidate for facelift surgery and the only thing that is holding you back is fear, I encourage you to read on and truly consider the facts. Facelift surgery is the gold standard in facial rejuvenation and can knock fifteen to twenty years off your appearance. You'll learn all you need to know about the realities of this procedure in Chapter 11.

11 Don't Fear the Facelift

More than any other procedure, people fear the facelift. Why are they so afraid? Most likely because they have seen how disastrous a facelift can be—the telltale scars; the strange, Joker-like proportions; the ears pinned to the sides of the face. How many Hollywood stars had a facelift and came out the other side unrecognizable? You might wonder, *If wealthy, powerful celebrities can't get it right, despite their access to the very best care, then how could I possibly look normal after a facelift?*

In fact, the facelift is the number one operation my patients fear. While they do not want to look older, neither do they want to look too "done" or "surgerized."

In addition to obvious or even garish results, many patients also fear the risks of anesthesia administered during facelifts. While some surgeons will perform facelifts only under general anesthesia, I perform them either under straight local anesthesia, with Novocain-like injections, or with twilight anesthetic, similar to what you might get during a colonoscopy if you choose to be asleep. Eighty percent of my patients opt for twilight, while 20 percent opt for local.

And yet, when done right, the facelift is a miraculously rejuvenating procedure. One technique in particular leaves the face appearing soft and smooth on the surface and avoids the dreaded, super-stretched, we-know-you-had-a-facelift look. It is called a deep plane facelift. I have published articles about this technique in peer-reviewed plastic surgery literature and presented on it at plastic surgery symposia all over the world. I have also lectured about it at the leading medical schools in the country, including Harvard, Yale, Stanford, Columbia, and the University of Pennsylvania. Hundreds of surgeons from all over the world have come to my office to witness me perform this technique and to learn how to make their own patients look just as sensational as mine. There is a simple reason for all of this: Deep plane facelifts really work, leaving my patients looking refreshed but still completely natural.

A deep plane facelift is the most timesaving and ultimately money-saving anti-aging procedure available. Here is a common story I hear from the people I treat. One of my favorite patients is a lovely woman who came to see me for fillers, Botox, and lasers for seven years, spending twice the cost of a surgery before she finally decided to have a deep plane facelift. After her surgery, she looked fifteen years younger but still exactly like herself (Figure 75). She regretted not having had the surgery earlier, not only because she would have looked

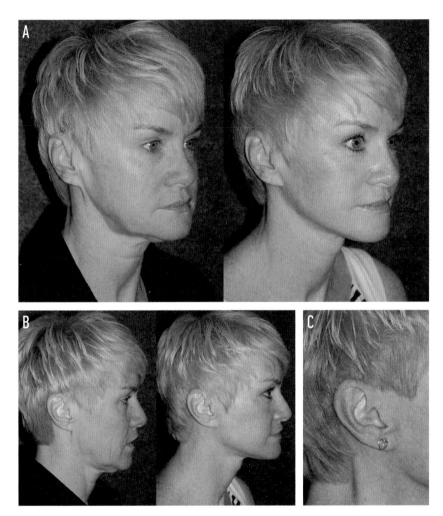

Figure 75: A, B) Before (left) and after (right) of a woman on whom I performed a minimal access deep plane extended (MADE) facelift. Notice natural tightening along the neck and jawline, as well as gentle lifting of the cheeks. She had been doing injectable fillers for years but finally decided for a more permanent fix. C) The close-up view of the ear shows the S-type incision is not visible.

so much better the last eight years but because she could have saved all that money. While a facelift isn't for everyone (and, depending on your age, it might be better to engage nonsurgical treatments before a facelift), understanding the ins and outs of the surgery will help you make the decision to pursue this option, or not, when the time comes. The most important thing I hope you'll learn from this chapter is that there is no reason to fear the facelift.

We will not be discussing nonsurgical facelifting in this chapter, as we covered liquid (filler) facelifts in Chapter 5 and energy-based devices to tighten the jawline and the neck in Chapter 10. The results from these procedures become more limited as aging progresses, which is often what brings patients to consider a facelift.

What Happens to Your Face as You Age

Many women will experience a rapid phase of facial aging in their late forties to early fifties; their faces will age more in two to three years than it had in the previous fifteen. The main cause of this is hormonal. In the late forties, women experience lower levels of estrogen and ultimately become perimenopausal. When this happens, the quality of the skin changes, and, within one to three years after becoming perimenopausal, the facial muscles loosen dramatically. Cheeks droop, creating folds between the nose and the corners of the mouth (nasolabial folds). Jowls form on either side of the chin, making this horizontal length of the lower face wider; and marionette lines or grooves develop between the corner of the mouth and chin. The descent of the cheeks and lower face make the face look chubbier. This is accompanied by neck laxity, which progresses to a "turkey gobbler," with vertical folds or bands developing in the neck.

While many people maintain the volume in their faces as they get older, some lose a significant amount, and their faces begin to look simultaneously gaunt and droopy. In these cases, the volume should be restored at the same time as the facelift is being performed, usually with fat grafting (see Chapter 5).

Surgical Facelift Procedures

For All Ethnicities

Facelifts can be overwhelming in part because there are so many names for different procedures: There are corporate-sponsored facelifts that are advertised on television, trade-marked lifts with interesting names for advertising and marketing purposes, mini lifts, S-lifts, MACS lifts, SMAS lifts, and deep plane lifts, to name just a few. This is all very confusing, and most people do not understand the inherent differences between techniques. How do you decide which procedure produces the best, longest-lasting results, with the least amount of scarring and healing downtime? It is important for patients to understand the pros and cons of different approaches so they can make an educated decision.

The three main facelift types are mini facelifts, SMAS facelifts, and deep plane facelifts. They all manipulate the musculature that droops with age, called the SMAS in the face and platysma in the neck, in different ways. SMAS, as discussed, is an acronym for the superficial musculo aponeurotic system, the layer of fibrous connective tissues (or fascia) and muscles that start just in front of and below the ear and extend down to the neck as the platysma. This thin yet strong layer covers and connects the muscles and structures of the face, the midface, and the neck together as a continuous fibro-muscular tissue. It encompasses areas of muscles, fat pads, and the entire cheek area. It also attaches to the superficial muscle that covers the lower face, the jawline, and neck muscles. The SMAS layer is covered superficially by a layer of fat and skin. The purpose of the SMAS is to ensure that the mimetic muscles, which allow you to make normal facial expressions, remain in place.

The information I provide in this chapter comes directly from my experience with all of these procedures, having performed thousands of facelifts throughout my career. I have arrived at performing the deep plane approach in the vast majority of my patients because of its superior natural rejuvenation and longer-lasting effects.

MINI FACELIFTS (SHORT SCAR AND S-LIFT)

A mini facelift is a popular method that rejuvenates the lower third of the face. It can also be called a short scar facelift or an S-lift. The term "S-lift" is derived from the shape of the smaller incision (like an "S"). It starts hidden in the sideburn hair, runs just inside the ear canal, and ends just behind the earlobe without running into the scalp skin behind the ear. A traditional facelift scar is usually twice as long, running up higher into the scalp above the ear and onto the scalp skin behind the ear. The S-lift does not distort the sideburns and hairline like more traditional facelifts. The S-lift incision

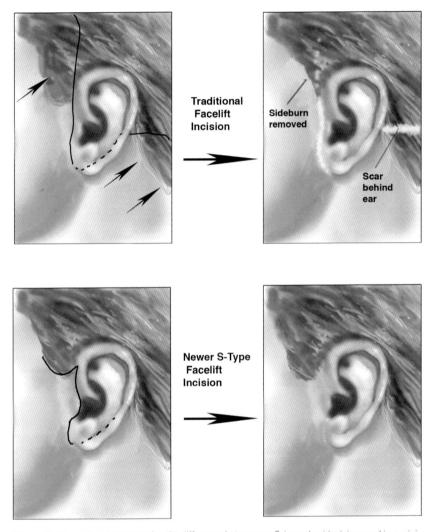

Traditional Facelift Incision

Sideburn removed

Scar behind ear

Newer S-Type Facelift Incision

Figure 76: Illustration demonstrating the difference between an S-type short incision used in a mini facelift and the incision used in a traditional facelift that is twice as long and not as well hidden.

is relatively well hidden; it is often called a "ponytail-type facelift" because you can put your hair up in a ponytail without having to worry about visible scars behind the ears (Figure 76).

The SMAS and the platysma are then tightened with stitches (called plication or imbrication sutures), but the SMAS is not elevated, as it would be in a traditional facelift. The jowls are corrected, but improvement in the neck is usually incomplete. This greater improvement in the face, when compared to the lack of change in the neck, looks ill matched, like the wrong lid on a jar. Because the muscles, which are the foundation of the face, are not lifted and resupported but simply stitched, the majority of the tightening is on the skin surface. This can leave patients with a windswept, stretched, or pulled appearance, as often seen in the dreaded West Coast style. Viewing these patients, it is easy to tell they've had work done—the corners of the mouth pulled, an obvious facelift giveaway. There is a lack of strength in the repair (of the muscles) of a mini lift, as it relies mostly on the relatively thin skin. Results last only three to five years.

What compounds this problem is that most facelifts, of all types, tighten the face toward the ears in a mostly horizontal direction. This is unnatural because the face falls vertically with gravity. Tightening horizontally across the face pulls the corners of the mouth, creating a "puppet mouth." Often the excess skin is also removed horizontally and the sideburns are cut away, another telltale sign of a facelift. All of this becomes difficult to hide and requires creative camouflaging with hairstyling, especially as you cannot wear your hair pulled back.

These problems can be avoided with a vertical vector facelift that I have pioneered. By lifting the face more vertically, a

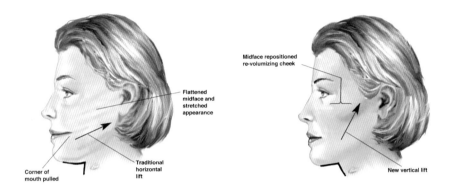

Figure 77: Illustration demonstrating how traditional facelifting (left) tightens the face horizontally, flattening the face and cheeks, leaving a "lifted" appearance, versus a vertical-oriented lift (right) that supports the cheeks, repositioning them upward. The vertical lift re-creates the "apple cheeks" of youth.

smoother and more natural appearance is created, the cheeks are restored, and the corners of the mouth that sag with age are elevated, not pulled. I performed clinical research to better define the angle of the proper direction of the facelift, finding that the ideal direction of the lift is 60 degrees for the average patient; I like to call this the "angle of maximal rejuvenation." Older patients require an angle of lift less than 60 degrees. Conversely, younger patients will require a more vertical facelift angle, often approaching 75 degrees (Figure 77).[1]

Although horizontal tightening can improve the jowls, it flattens the cheeks, exaggerating their deflated appearance. The nasolabial folds remain unchanged. Because of the lack of cheek improvement with this technique, many doctors will also incorporate fat transfers (as described in Chapter 5). This can be effective if performed well, but fat transfers have two downsides:

1. If the cheeks were not lifted vertically and fat is stacked on top of the descended cheeks, the face will look overly full.
2. Fat transfers reabsorb in a third of cases and are often not permanent.

SMAS FACELIFTS

The main differences between mini facelifts and SMAS facelifts are the incision and the amount of work done to the underlying muscle of the face. SMAS lifts usually have a longer incision that continues onto the scalp skin behind the ear to allow more work on the neck. After the skin is lifted, the SMAS muscles in the lower face along the jowl region and the platysma muscle in the neck are lifted (as opposed to being simply stitched together), giving the face more support. SMAS techniques do not lift the cheeks because the SMAS muscle ends at the outer border of the cheek musculature (called the zygomaticus musculature). With better neck results, these lifts have been shown to last around eight to ten years. They still suffer from a lack of improvement in the cheeks, since SMAS lifts also horizontally tighten the face. There are "high SMAS" and "low SMAS" variations of this procedure that are beyond the scope of this book, but they both have the same limitations. In a SMAS facelift, the skin is separated from the muscle, so it still has a tendency to appear tighter or "plastic" on the surface, but less so than with a mini facelift that provides less support to the muscles.

DEEP PLANE AND MINIMAL ACCESS DEEP PLANE EXTENDED (MADE) FACELIFTS

The deep plane facelift avoids the problem of the tight, over-filled look of many modern West Coast–style facelifts. The main tenet of the deep plane facelift is that it lifts only under the muscle layer, leaving the skin attached to the muscle, so it can never look tight. It also lifts the cheeks by releasing the tethering points of the face in the deep plane so that the addition of fat or filler is unnecessary.

The "deep plane" is the term used to describe the anatomic plane that exists between the SMAS-platysma complex (which is muscle and fascia) and the deeper layer of muscles responsible for facial expression. The deep plane facelift focuses on release and movement of muscle and fat layers, instead of skin pull and removal. The extended deep plane facelift that I have developed incorporates the release of the ligaments tethering the deep plane layer to achieve tension-free movement so that no tightness is created by the facelift procedure. There are four ligaments that I release with corresponding natural lifting throughout the face and neck (Figure 78), all of which I'll describe in this chapter. While this information may be fairly technical, I think it is important to understand the mechanics that prevent the bad facelift outcomes feared by most patients who are considering the procedure. Since the deeper layer used in a deep plane facelift is fibrous and inelastic, unlike the skin, which is very elastic, the deep plane facelift procedure has the most long-lasting results of any facelifting technique.

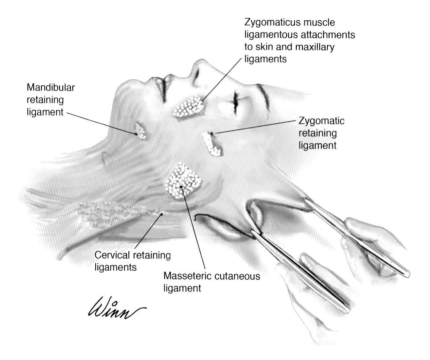

Zygomaticus muscle
ligamentous attachments
to skin and maxillary
ligaments

Mandibular
retaining
ligament

Zygomatic
retaining
ligament

Cervical retaining
ligaments

Masseteric cutaneous
ligament

Winn

Figure 78: The extended deep plane facelift incorporates the release of four facial ligaments tethering the deep plane layer to achieve tension-free movement so that no tightness is created by the facelift procedure.

The first ligaments released are the zygomatic ligaments that tether the cheek so that they can be elevated superiorly. Releasing the zygomatic ligaments restores the cheek shape and volume, re-creating the heart-shaped face of youth; releasing these ligaments removes the need to add filler, fat, or cheek implants to the face. It also improves the nasolabial folds and the hollowing and shadowing seen under the lower eyelids by restoring volume that is lost to gravitational descent associated with aging. I have published research in the *Aesthetic Surgery Journal* showing that this restores cheek volume equivalent to adding three vials of injected filler into each cheek.[2] The cost

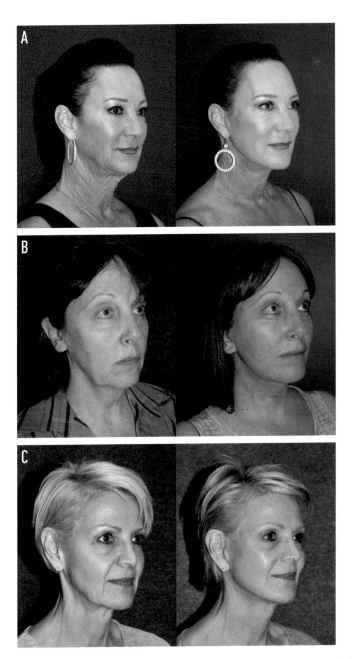

Figure 79: A, B, C) Before (left) and after (right) of three women on whom I performed a MADE facelift. Notice how elevating the cheek muscle and fat compartments vertically re-creates the heart shape of youth and restores the cheek volume without adding fillers or fat to the cheeks.

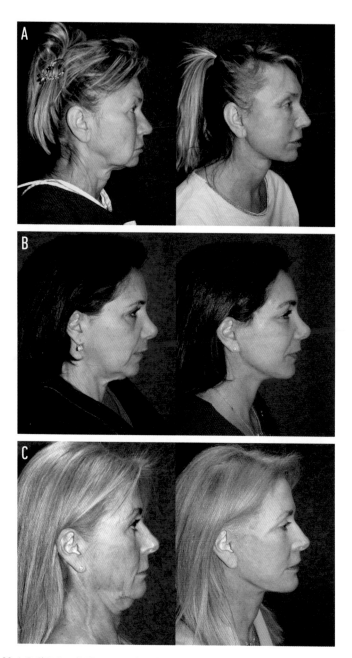

Figure 80: A, B, C) Before (left) and after (right) of three women on whom I performed a MADE facelift. Notice how releasing the retaining ligaments along the jawline allows for tension-free smoothing along the jowls, creating an unoperated youthful jawline. A) She also had fractional laser resurfacing and a lateral temporal brow lift at the same time. C) She also had a lip lift.

of six vials of hyaluronic acid filler is $6,000 in most practices in New York City, and the filler will reabsorb within one year (Figure 79).

Even though the deep plane facelift helps restore facial shape and repositions cheek fat, there are patients who require additional volume augmentation. If you are very thin or have more sunken cheeks, fat grafting (as described in Chapter 5) is necessary to perform at the same time as the facelift.

The next two ligaments that are released are the masseteric and mandibular ligaments. They tether the jowl, and releasing them allows me to create a smooth and crisp jawline appearance without it appearing tight (Figure 80).

The fourth and last ligament that is released is the cervical retaining ligament that tethers the hanging platysma muscle in the neck. A common problem in facelifting is early failure of the neck lift portion of the operation, with neck skin hanging again after a few years. To combat this problem, I was one of the first surgeons to describe the release of the cervical retaining ligaments in the neck so that it can be lifted more durably.[3] This allows for more significant re-draping of the drooping neck muscles, which means that the rejuvenation and refinement in the neck and jawline are more natural and longer lasting. This part of the technique also improves the definition along the angle of the jaw (you may remember the gonial angle from Chapter 9), which is often blunted by bunching that is created in SMAS techniques (Figure 81).

I understand that patients are worried about scarring, so I have created a technique that combines the benefits of the deep

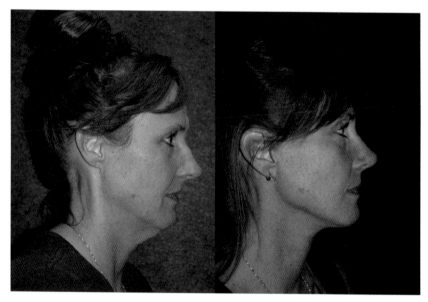

Figure 81: Before (left) and after (right) of a woman on whom I performed a MADE facelift. Notice how lifting on the deep neck muscles and not stretching the skin allows for a smooth neckline that looks youthful, not tight.

plane procedure with the short incision technique. This hybrid deep plane facelift I pioneered is called a minimal access deep plane extended (MADE) facelift. Using endoscopes, I can work through these smaller incisions. These smaller incisions are the S-type "minimal access." I have published this technique in the *Aesthetic Surgery Journal* and have performed it on about a thousand patients.[4]

Depending on the degree of neck drooping and heaviness that occurs, the deep plane facelift may be combined with a corset platysmaplasty (described in Chapter 10). Through a small hidden incision under the chin, vertical cords and bands in the neck can be tightened and the chin fat that accumulates with age can be removed. Because the extended deep plane facelift lifts the platysma more significantly than other facelifting techniques, the additional midline surgery, trauma, and recovery associated with facelifts can be avoided in a majority of cases.

Patients who wish to stop smoking (and I encourage all of my patients to stop smoking, since it's not only bad for general health but dangerous for surgical procedures) have to do so cold turkey, because nicotine patches are as bad for the surgery as actively smoking. Interestingly, deep plane lifts are the only facelift type that can be performed safely on smokers. The nicotine in cigarettes causes the blood vessels in the skin to narrow. If the skin is separated from the muscle as described in SMAS and mini lifts, it can necrose or die, resulting in weeks of healing and bad scars. However, I have performed studies showing that deep plane lifts can be performed safely in smokers, as the skin and muscle are not separated, preserving the blood supply to the lifted tissues.

ENDOSCOPIC MIDFACE LIFTS

For those patients who do not require any improvement of the jawline and neck, there is a minimally invasive surgical procedure to lift the drooped cheeks called an endoscopic midface lift. This is most commonly performed on women and men in their forties to early fifties.

Endoscopic midface lifts use only two small incisions hidden in the hairline, just big enough to allow the insertion of an endoscope the size of a drinking straw. The deep tissues, including the muscles and cheek fat pad called the malar fat

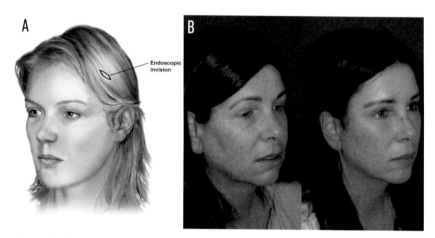

Figure 82: A) Illustration showing the incision used to perform an endoscopic midface lift to lift the cheeks and central portions of the face. There is no scarring, as the incision is hidden inside the hairline. B) Before (left) and after (right) of a patient who had an endoscopic midface lift to re-create the heart-shaped face of youth by lifting the cheeks.

pad, are lifted off the cheekbones and repositioned vertically, and permanent sutures are placed that suspend them to the muscles in the temples. This procedure has the advantage of shorter incisions and a shorter recovery than the facelifts described above and should last between five and seven years (Figure 82). Imagine a line drawn from the corner of the mouth to the ear canal. This procedure rejuvenates all of the drooping tissues above this line but not below it. I find that many of my patients want further tightening along the lower face and jawline, even if they do not want their neck lifted. In these cases, a MADE facelift would actually be the best option.

UNIQUE CHARACTERISTICS FOR ASIAN FACELIFTS

I am always happy to work on patients who have come to me from all over the world, including from China, Korea, Japan,

Thailand, and Singapore. Asian patients age differently than other ethnicities. I often see that they come for a facelift consult ten years later than Caucasians because their faces droop more slowly. Their thicker skin does not descend as readily or show fine wrinkles as early. Other unique characteristics of the Asian face include a flatter facial skeleton and denser, larger zygomatic (cheek) ligaments. They have heavier tissues that accumulate more fat in the buccal or cheek fat pads and lower face and neck area as they age. Because of this, volume in the cheeks and neckline needs to be reduced. This is often the opposite of what happens to most Caucasian faces, where volume loss requires the supplementation of fat grafting during facelifting.

To correct these problems, a facelift that focuses on the deeper structure, musculature, and fat planes of the face is important—more superficial facelifts will not correct these issues. SMAS facelifts are less effective on Asian patients because they do not release their strong cheek ligaments, so the face cannot be adequately lifted and tightened. The deep plane facelift lifts the deeper structure of the face to support the thicker and heavier tissues of the Asian face and so will last longer term. It also allows access to the buccal fat pads of the cheeks and neck fat, which often require reduction. Accordingly, I often suggest the deep plane approach to my Asian patients (Figure 83).

Asian patients also have the tendency to develop hypertrophic scarring and keloid scars much more frequently than patients of other ethnicities. Deep plane facelifts help avoid this problem. With its deeply supported lift under the muscles, there is no tension or pulling on the incision lines once closed.

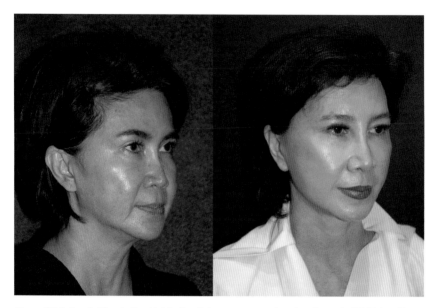

Figure 83: Before (left) and after (right) of an Asian woman on whom I performed a MADE facelift. The deep plane approach is better for Asian faces as they have heavier facial tissues and broader facial ligaments that require more extensive facial lifting to create long-lasting results.

This tension-free closure allows the incision to heal as imperceptible fine lines. As an additional measure of caution, the scar is hidden inside the tragus (a cartilage of the ear canal) so that it cannot be seen.

UNIQUE CHARACTERISTICS FOR AFRICAN AMERICAN FACELIFTS

African Americans have skin that is extremely thin, with amazing elasticity—this is why they wrinkle less than Caucasians as they get older. Similar to Asians, their faces show signs of aging a decade later than most Caucasians. Their aging shows up mostly in the areas of the neck that begin to droop, as well as in the jawline and drooping jowls.

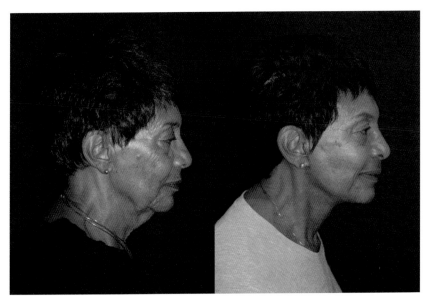

Figure 84: Before (left) and after (right) of an African American woman on whom I performed a MADE facelift. African American skin requires different techniques to prevent scarring and change in skin color.

The big issue for African American patients is potential scarring (as with Asian patients). As described previously, tension-free closure with the deep plane technique allows incisions to heal as imperceptible fine lines, so that hypertrophic or keloid scarring can be avoided (Figure 84).

African American patients do have a few additional risks. There is a higher risk for both hyperpigmentation (darkening of the skin) and hypopigmentation (lightening of the skin) after surgery. These problems can be treated with topical hydro-quinone creams, but vigilance is required, and early treatment helps mitigate these problems. When compared to other ethnicities, African Americans have roughly a 40 percent higher risk of heart disease and a 60 percent higher risk for diabetes, so pre-operative testing is a must. These health conditions can affect healing after surgery.

FACELIFTS FOR MEN

In male plastic surgery, any appearance of tightness to the face is unacceptable, as it can feminize the face. The appearance of tightness across the beard line can also look manipulated. My Park Avenue patients must look like themselves after surgery; they are CEOs, hedge fund managers, lawyers, and professionals, and their faces are their calling cards. A West Coast–style tight face could be career-ending.

Early in my career, when I performed SMAS facelifts regularly, even lifting the SMAS muscle, there was always a resulting hint of tightness across the face that could be picked up

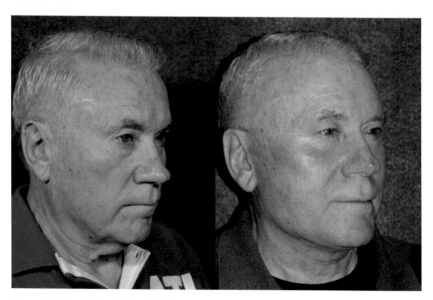

Figure 85: Before (left) and after (right) of a male patient on whom I performed a MADE facelift. The deep plane facelift lifts the male face, leaving no tension on the surface so it does not feminize the face.

by a more sophisticated observer. This simply does not happen after deep plane facelift surgery. As described earlier, deep plane surgery does not peel the skin away from the muscles, so that the skin cannot appear tight or stretched. Lifting under the muscle layer alone leaves the surface soft and natural (Figure 85). Recently, I performed a face and neck lift on a sixty-year-old hedge fund manager who went on rounds of fundraising meetings in Europe just two weeks after his surgery. He went with his business partner, who is the same age. At a dinner meeting, the forty-year-old investor to whom they were pitching their business mistakenly assumed that my patient was also forty, even going so far as to remark, "When we get to be your partner's age in twenty years, we better have our retirement plans set."

For men, hidden incisions are all the more important, since most wear short hair (or are bald). The incisions can be completely hidden inside the ear canal and behind the ear so that even if you do not have hair on your head, no one will be able to tell you've had surgery. One thing to be aware of is that when the extra skin is removed, the bearded skin is moved into the incision in your ear canal, so additional grooming for the extra hair growing inside your ear will be required. I suggest getting a small electronic trimmer for grooming nasal and ear hair.

Men tend to bleed more during surgery because their bearded faces have more blood supply than women's. Men have a higher rate of hematomas (blood collecting under the tissues) after surgery than women and develop more bruising.

I tell my male patients they need at least two weeks away from the office to recover.

BOTCHED FACELIFTS: WHAT CAN GO WRONG AND HOW TO FIX IT

There are many reasons people seek revision facelifts. One scenario is the patient has had a successful facelift, but it has naturally aged over time and a new surgery is required to maintain his or her youthful appearance. In general, well-performed facelifts last more than ten years. It's also possible that a person has had a facelift and the result was not acceptable because areas of the face were under-treated. The most common problems include continued jowls or neck laxity after surgery or drooping of the cheeks and mid-facial area. Procedures that do not last as long as anticipated are also a very common reason a person will inquire about a secondary facelift. The most common cause of under-correction and shorter-term results is when a surgeon employs a more superficial-based facelift technique. I see this problem regularly in my practice, not only because I specialize in revising facelift surgery but because more than 90 percent of plastic surgeons perform superficial-based facelifts, simply placing sutures on the surface of the facial muscles, achieving limited results. They do not lift the supportive musculature of the face (the SMAS muscle in the cheek and platysma muscle in the neck). A deep plane facelift is the answer to this problem.

Then there is the patient whose face looks irregular after a facelift and who wants more surgery to normalize his or her appearance. The three most common problems caused by botched surgery are the overdone "stretched face," poor scarring around the ears with loss of hair (sideburns) and hairline distortions, and a strange neck appearance called the cobra neck deformity (described in Chapter 10).

First, let's address the "stretched face," which is seen on far too many patients, whether they prefer the West Coast or the East Coast style. This result tends to be most problematic for those patients with thinner skin and requires special treatment to avoid further complications from a secondary facelift. This tightness on the surface of the skin creates what doctors call a "lateral sweep deformity," because of the characteristic sweeping lines across the sides of the face caused by too much superficial tension on the skin and by pulling the SMAS and skin laterally or toward the ears (Figure 86).

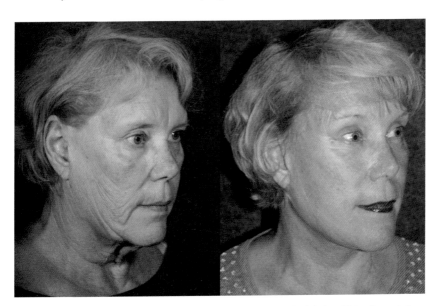

Figure 86: Before (left) and after (right) of a woman who had an overly tight facelift (performed elsewhere), on whom I performed a corrective deep plane facelift. By supporting the deep facial muscles, tension is taken off the skin surface so that the stretched face looks smooth again.

I have published my technique for dealing with this problem because I do so many revision facelifts in my practice.[5] During some weeks, revisions can comprise up to 30 percent of the facelifts I perform. This overly tight and stretched face is best treated with a deep plane technique to relieve the tension from the surface of the skin and lift the face vertically. Because patients who wind up with this problem often have thin skin, they also often require multilevel fat transfers and grafting to thicken the skin and restore facial volume.

Obvious scars and ear and hairline distortions will also give away the fact that you had a bad facelift. To hide these problems, wearing the hair down is necessary, or if you are a man or woman who likes to wear your hair short, you will need to grow it. When the skin is too tight on closure of the facelift, it

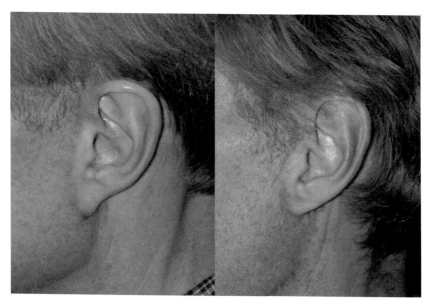

Figure 87: Before (left) and after (right) of corrective plastic surgery to fix a "pixie ear deformity" in which the earlobes got elongated after an overly tight facelift.

not only makes the surface stretch, it causes the scars to widen and become thick (what doctors call a hypertrophic scar). This pulling also causes the earlobes to stretch and elongate into a pattern called a "pixie ear deformity" (Figure 87). Unfortunately, performing a scar revision will not fix this. Cutting out the scar and attempting to reposition the earlobe will only create more tension on the new incision line; the scarring will re-form and the earlobe will pull down again. Instead, a revision facelift that supports the skin at the muscle level is required. Executing a deep plane facelift will take the tension off the skin and will result in no tension or pulling on the incision lines once closed. This tension-free closure allows the incision to heal as imperceptible fine lines, and the muscles will support the earlobes and prevent them from pulling down once again.

A "cobra neck" deformity, which we also discussed in Chapter 10, is an odd, surgerized contour in the neck created during facelifting. In this situation, the center of the neck is caved in and there is hanging of the neck and jowls on either side, creating a shape similar to a cobra snake's head. This problem occurs when too much tissue is removed from the center of the neck from overaggressive liposuction during surgery, and the neck platysma muscles are not tightened in the center of the neck. Simple mini facelifts can create this problem because they do minimal muscle tightening, attempting to tighten the neck with liposuction to remove fat from the neck. The only way to correct this problem is with a corset platysmaplasty that elevates the hanging pieces on either side of the neck and tightens them in the midline, reducing the sides of the cobra head and transferring the muscle volume to the gouged-out area in the center of the neck. Occasionally, if further volume correction is required, fat transfers, with fat suctioned from other parts of the body, can be added.

Facial nerve injury is the most dreaded complication of facelifting. This is when one or more branches of the facial nerve are weakened from the facelift surgery, and it affects the ability of the patient to animate or express the face. When you smile, the corner of the mouth will elevate on one side more than the other and can look crooked. Facelifts can result in temporary (lasting around six weeks) or permanent facial nerve weaknesses. The rate of temporary weakness is 1 percent, which means it does not happen 99 percent of the time; it is self-limiting and resolves spontaneously. Temporary facial nerve weakness results from bruising that occurs after surgery and is not due to any problem with the facelift technique or how it was performed. The rate of temporary facial nerve injury is the same for all facelifting techniques, whether superficial or deep plane. Permanent facial nerve injuries are extremely rare and have been reported to happen in one in ten thousand facelifts performed (you are more likely to get in a fatal car accident than experience permanent facial nerve injury after surgery). There are procedures to repair a facial nerve injury that require microsurgery, but due to the extreme rarity of this problem and the complex nature of the repairs, which are difficult to explain, I will not discuss them here.

What to Expect After Facelift Surgery

Recovery following a deep plane facelift usually involves some bruising and swelling around the repositioned areas for the first few days. These symptoms will gradually disappear. Because the deep plane technique is accomplished in the layer that naturally exists in our face, there is minimal bruising and minimal pain after the procedure. Deep plane surgery also maintains more of the natural blood supply to the skin by not severing blood vessels between the muscle and skin, allowing for more rapid healing. SMAS facelifts lift under the skin, disrupting blood vessels, and thus result in greater bruising.

Pain medication may be prescribed to help the patient to feel more comfortable during the healing process. Interestingly, there is very little pain after facelift surgery, since it causes the area around the incisions and the face to go numb for six weeks. That means the area affected will not have any sensation to touch, but it will move normally. The center of the face (your nose, lips, and eyes) will feel normal. In the beginning, numbing will feel like a blessing, but as time goes on, most patients find it odd and anxiously await the return of sensation to their faces. I encourage my patients to apply cold compresses to help alleviate swelling and recommend elevation of the head. It is important to get plenty of rest during the recovery.

Deep plane facelift incisions heal with minimal to no visible scarring. Because the deep plane facelift does not separate the skin and the lift is supported under the muscles, there is no tension or pulling on the incision lines once closed. This tension-free closure allows the incision to heal as impercepti-ble fine lines. It also prevents any pulling of the earlobe after facelift, which can create a "pixie ear."

While, as with any surgery, a facelift can involve risks and challenges, the truth is that these procedures are largely safe, producing some of the most transformative results possible in the world of facial plastic surgery. There is no reason to fear the facelift—especially after reading this guide. You know what to look for, what questions to ask, and what to expect at every stage of any process you decide to pursue. It's an incredible time to be a patient, with cutting-edge technological advances revolutionizing surgical and nonsurgical procedures, and if you are ready, there is no reason to wait to do something about the problem that has bothered you for years. When you look good, you feel good.

The Park Avenue Face is *your* face, just as natural and unique, only younger, more balanced, more defined. You are now well equipped to make informed decisions about your doctor and your procedure, and it's this knowledge that makes all the dif-ference when it comes to the success of facial plastic surgery. So, what's stopping you from being your best you?

1 Andrew A. Jacono and Evan R. Ransom, "Patient-Specific Rhytidectomy: Finding the Angle of Maximal Rejuvenation," *Aesthetic Surgery Journal* 32, no. 7 (2012), 804–813, doi: 10.1177/1090820X12455826, https://academic.oup.com/asj/article/32/7/804/220126.

2 Andrew A. Jacono, Melanie H. Malone, and Ben Talei, "Three-Dimensional Analysis of Long-Term Midface Volume Change After Vertical Vector Deep-Plane Rhytidectomy," *Aesthetic Surgery Journal* 35, no. 5 (2015), 491–503, doi: 10.1093/asj/sju171, https://www.ncbi.nlm.nih.gov/pubmed/26063830.

3 Andrew A. Jacono and Melanie H. Malone, "Characterization of the Cervical Retaining Ligaments During Subplatysmal Facelift Dissection and its Implications," *Aesthetic Surgery Journal* 37, no. 5 (2017), 495–501, doi: 10.1093/asj/sjw274, https://www.ncbi.nlm.nih.gov/pubmed/28200084.

4 Andrew A. Jacono and Suchita S. Parikh, "The Minimal Access Deep Plane Extended Vertical Facelift," *Aesthetic Surgery Journal* 31, no. 8 (2011), 874–890, doi: 10.1177/1090820X11424146, https://www.ncbi.nlm.nih.gov/pubmed/22065880.

5 Andrew A. Jacono and Melanie H. Malone, "Vertical Sweep Deformity After Face-lift," *JAMA Facial Plastic Surgery* 19, no. 2 (2017), 155–156, doi: 10.1001/jamafacial.2016.1602, https://www.ncbi.nlm.nih.gov/pubmed/28006056.

12 Anesthesia and Healing

Today, there are more anesthesia and healing options than there were even five years ago. These, coupled with advancements in minimally invasive anti-aging techniques, have allowed us to experience a golden age in the field of facial plastic surgery. Patients no longer need to worry about the risks associated with general anesthesia, nor do they have to spend two weeks hiding out after a facelift. In the age of customization as luxury, I'm happy to report that facial plastic surgery is at the forefront of this trend. From multiple anesthesia options to homeopathic healing and hyperbaric oxygen treatments, you have the ability to tailor your facial rejuvenation experience to exactly what fits your goals and lifestyle.

Anesthesia: General or Local?

Every day in my practice I am asked by patients whether their surgery can be performed without general anesthesia. General anesthesia involves being paralyzed during surgery with medications administered by an anesthesiologist, including placement of a breathing tube and breathing anesthetic gas. Patients are concerned about the risks involved with having general anesthesia because it puts a significant amount of strain on the body. Other patients have experienced days of feeling ill with nausea, headaches, and weakness after general anesthesia, and they want to avoid it at all costs.

My answer to them is that we rarely use general anesthesia in my practice when performing facial plastic surgery. In fact, unless it is necessary because the patient has some other medical condition that requires it, I prefer not to use it. General anesthetic drugs and gases cause major physiologic changes in the body; they cause blood vessels to dilate, increasing how much you bleed during surgery. This causes bruising and swelling, which increases recovery time. Additionally, general anesthesia can induce vomiting, which can lead to further trauma and torn sutures for some patients.

I also employ music therapy prior to injections and during the local anesthesia surgery. It has been shown that playing relaxing music that a patient prefers helps lower a patient's blood pressure during surgery. This limits bleeding, and therefore minimizes bruising.

For patients who do not want to be awake and aware during surgery, I use a twilight anesthesia. This is called propofol,

You Don't Need General Anesthesia to Have Plastic Surgery!

When I perform surgery on patients, I give them different options for their anesthesia, because it is not a one-size-fits-all approach. I either perform it under a local anesthesia, which means the patient is wide awake and has surgery after numbing shots are administered, or under a twilight anesthesia given through an IV (no anesthesia gas is given) where the patient is asleep and not aware. In my practice, only 20 percent of my patients do surgery wide awake under a local anesthetic, and 80 percent of patients have a twilight anesthetic where they are asleep for the surgery, but in *neither* case are they under general anesthesia.

Eyelid lifts, rhinoplasties, lip augmentation surgery, chin and cheek augmentation, facelifts, and many other procedures can be easily and safely performed under local anesthesia. This means being given a minor sedative such as Valium in a pill form to relax you, after which your plastic surgeon injects Novocain-like local shots (similar to the ones you would get at the dentist) to numb the part of the face having surgery. I use drugs called Lidocaine and Marcaine because they last longer and are more effective than Novocain. The shots can be painful and multiple shots need to be administered, but we use a tiny needle that spreads the medicine slowly to minimize discomfort. Because of this discomfort, I do not suggest this procedure for those who are afraid of needles or have a very low pain threshold. The value in local anesthesia is that it decreases the amount of bleeding during surgery when compared to general anesthesia, and therefore bruising and post-operative recovery time are lessened. Also, the surgeon gives the shots to numb the face, which saves the patient money by eliminating the need for an anesthesiologist.

the same anesthesia given intravenously during a colonoscopy. This medication is like an intravenous Valium, but as soon as the medicine is turned off, you wake up in a few minutes, without any nausea or hangover headache from general anesthesia gas. Twilight anesthesia also reduces bruising compared to general anesthesia. It is extremely safe, and patients often feel great after surgery, just as if they had a restful night's sleep. Any person who has had a colonoscopy (and I am one of them) can attest to this fact.

One way I modify a twilight type of anesthesia is in rhinoplasty cases. During a rhinoplasty, I place a dam in the back of the throat called an LMA that prevents blood from dripping into the windpipe. Because you are sleeping you cannot protect your airway, which can become blocked with a blood clot. This does not happen under local anesthesia because an awake "nose job" patient can swallow and clear the blood away with a hand-held suction tube during surgery. This is an important modification that I suggest any patient discuss with their surgeon prior to having a rhinoplasty surgery under twilight anesthesia.

Many plastic surgeons will only perform surgery under general anesthesia. While I do agree that the risks of having serious complications after anesthesia are extremely low (less than .001 percent), there is no question that the rate of nausea, discomfort, and the increased bruising associated with general anesthesia warrant these surgeons reconsider their approach. In my opinion, the reason why surgeons continue to do surgery exclusively under general anesthesia has more to do with the doctor's comfort in performing surgery with the patient in this state than with the best option for the patient.

Pre-Surgery Dos and Don'ts

Faster healing time is among the top concerns of facial plastic surgery patients because they are all very busy and are eager to return to their public lives as quickly as possible. Until recently, patients desiring a younger or aesthetically more balanced look have had to submit to a procedure such as a facelift that required a two- to three-week recovery and a risk of visible scarring. As you know from previous chapters, one way to minimize recovery is to seek out a highly skilled facial plastic surgeon who employs minimal incision approaches and less traumatic techniques, which reduce recovery time.

As important as the surgeon you choose is how you prepare for your surgery. All patients should have a complete physical examination by their internist (not their plastic surgeon) to assess their physical wellness and preparedness for surgery. A simple example is that poorly controlled high blood pressure can result in excessive bleeding after surgery and hence more bruising and swelling. Medications that are prescribed by your physician that will thin the blood or inhibit surgical healing should be substituted.

With this completed, I start my patients on a strict regimen two weeks prior to surgery. The first thing patients must do is avoid medications, supplements, and habits that reduce the body's ability to stop bleeding during surgery, which will inevitably increase post-procedure bruising, swelling, and recovery time. These medications, supplements, and habits may include:

- **Aspirin, Plavix, Coumadin, and anti-inflammatories** (over-the-counter drugs such as Advil, Motrin, Aleve, Naproxen) either impair platelet function or protein production necessary for clotting. Be aware that most cold remedies contain these drugs. Tylenol (acetaminophen) is the only safe painkiller in the pre-operative period.
- **Vitamin E** can thin the blood and cause more bleeding and bruising. Many health foods, shakes, and energy bars have excessive Vitamin E.
- **Omega-3s and fish oils** are wonderful nutritional supplements, but they can inhibit clotting and increase bleeding during surgery.
- **Ginko biloba** has an anti-coagulant affect and causes bleeding.
- **Willow bark** is an herbal supplement that contains salicin, which is a precursor of aspirin.
- **Smoking** increases swelling, limits blood flow to the skin during healing, and worsens scarring. If you

smoke, you need to refrain from smoking two weeks before and two weeks after surgery. That means no nicotine for one month, including no nicotine gums to curb cravings as nicotine is the culprit that affects healing. Due to the difficulty of the task, I often give patients a prescriptive medicine such as Chantix that helps them kick the habit short term. There is a light at the end of the tunnel for smokers, as they can return to this destructive habit. What is wonderful is that patients will often stop smoking permanently after surgery; the surgery was the catalyst to cessation. There is a dual benefit in this situation: Not only are you healthier but the surgical procedure will last longer in a nonsmoker—about twice as long.

- **Alcohol** intake should be avoided completely for two weeks before surgery, as it also will thin the blood.

There are other "housekeeping" items to address within two weeks of surgery. For patients who color their hair, do so as close as possible to the date of surgery, as you cannot dye the hair again until four weeks after surgery. All medication needed after surgery should be purchased and at home before surgery. All post-operative instruction sheets should be reviewed and available at home to refer back to after surgery. Do not eat after midnight the day before surgery, as it will delay the procedure. Finally, wear a comfortable outfit to surgery, usually a sweat suit with a shirt that zips or buttons down the front so that it will not be necessary to pull it over the face after your procedure.

Homeopathic Healing and Hyperbaric Oxygen

Now that your body has been prepared for the surgery, there are three major ways to increase the recovery of facial plastic surgery during and after the surgery. During the surgery, one should avoid general anesthesia because it results in dilation of blood vessels, leading to more bleeding during surgery and more bruising after surgery. After the surgery, homeopathic and nutritional supplements that have been proven in clinical studies to improve healing should be introduced to your diet. Hyperbaric oxygen therapy treatments can be incorporated post-operatively due to their ability to speed healing.

Homeopathy is a system of natural healthcare that has been in worldwide use for more than two hundred years. It is recognized by the World Health Organization as the second-largest therapeutic system in use in the world. While it is most popular in India and South America, more than 30 million people in Europe and millions of others around the world also benefit from its use.

I have been prescribing homeopathic remedies to my own patients for years. What I have found to be most difficult is for my patients to find the exact supplements and homeopathic treatments at their local health food store, let alone find them at the correct strengths and formulations.

That is why I created the J Pak Systems. J Pak Systems is a homeopathic healing supplement system that provides an all-in-one, convenient solution featuring precise doses of the most refined, concentrated, bio-available formulas in single-dose packets. J Pak No. 1 is for use before and after

Natural Remedies for the Win

Homeopathy is founded on the principle of "like cures like." The body knows what it is doing, and symptoms are the body's way of taking action to overcome illness. This healing response is automatic in living organisms. The similar medicine acts as a stimulus to the natural vital response, giving it the information it needs to complete its healing work. Scientific studies indicate that homeopathic remedies such as Arnica montana and dietary supplements such as bromelain and hyaluronic acid can help minimize swelling and bruising and speed healing.

aesthetic injectable treatments to minimize bruising and swelling, and J Pak No. 2 is for use after plastic surgery to optimize healing.

Both J Pak No. 1 and J Pak No. 2 contain arnica and bromelain. Arnica montana, or leopard's bane, is a perennial herb indigenous to central Europe that has long been used to reduce post-traumatic bruising and swelling. Published studies indicate that Arnica montana can significantly reduce bruising and swelling. Bromelain is an enzyme derived from pineapple stems with anti-inflammatory properties. Published studies indicate that bromelain reduced edema (swelling) and ecchymosis (bruising) following surgical and nonsurgical trauma to the face.

J Pak No. 2 contains other nutritional supplements required for healing, including hyaluronic acid, glucosamine, vitamin C, and zinc. The regimen is started three days before surgery to get the body fueled for the healing process and then continued for two weeks post-surgery. Hyaluronic acid is a carbohydrate component of the extracellular (outside the cells) matrix of skin and is secreted during wound and tissue repair. It is produced by fibroblasts (cells in the skin) during wound repair. Published studies indicate that hyaluronic acid helps accelerate healing. Glucosamine compounds have been reported to have several beneficial effects on the skin and its cells. Because glucosamine stimulates hyaluronic acid synthesis, it has also been shown to accelerate wound healing, improve skin hydration, and decrease wrinkles. Vitamin C is an essential cofactor for collagen production and wound healing, which requires the production of new collagen. Zinc is an essential trace element in the human body. It serves as a cofactor in skin cell migration during wound repair.

Whether you are having noninvasive or more invasive treatments to enhance your facial appearance, the J Pak Systems can help speed your recovery so you can start enjoying your results earlier. J Pak Systems products can be purchased at www.jpaksystems.com.

Up until now, homeopathy was the only way to increase the speed of healing and get back to work and your social life more quickly. I performed a study to identify whether hyperbaric oxygen (HBO) therapy would increase how quickly my patients heal. HBO works to increase oxygen to facial tissue and stimulate the growth of new blood vessels, which, in turn, contributes to a faster recovery.[1] In this study, patients underwent HBO therapy for two days before their facelift surgery and three days after surgery. The study showed that hyperbaric oxygen decreases bruising by 35 percent at one week after surgery. Hyperbaric oxygen therapy offers patients an additional option for quicker recovery from facelift surgery and potentially other cosmetic procedures. It is an excellent tool for patients with limited available recovery time for faster resolution of post-operative swelling and bruising.

---

1 Andrew A. Jacono and Benjamin C. Stong, "Effect of Perioperative Hyperbaric Oxygen on Bruising in Face-Lifts," *Archives of Facial Plastic Surgery* 12, no. 5 (2010), 356–358, doi: 10.1001/archfacial.2010.66, https://www.ncbi.nlm.nih.gov/pubmed/20855782.

Conclusion

Do you feel better about your options for plastic surgery now? I hope so!

Even in our social media–driven era of digitally enhanced images, my patients come to know that there is no such thing as a perfect face—only the face that is perfect for their wants and needs. My job is to inform them of all the incredible options available to them and to give them the best possible results that fit their budget and their schedules, and, most of all, the results that will enhance the natural beauty they already possess. That's why I've written this book!

Whether you call the East Coast or the West Coast style your own, whether you are driven or define yourself by the cult of youth or by the cult of success, a little bit of due diligence will make you the savviest shopper for the best possible procedure. Some of my patients may want only a few Botox shots and an occasional injection of a filler, and that makes them totally happy. Others may go right for the deep plane (MADE) facelift, wanting to look as rejuvenated and refreshed as possible, with minimal pain and downtime. Some may want to share the results with everyone they know, while others will *never* admit to having had "a little work." Some may want to be knocked out completely with the most potent anesthesia on the market, while others are thrilled that I offer them the option of having local anesthesia only (even for a facelift!)

because to them it's worth the sting of a few needles to have a shorter recovery time.

Whatever procedure you are considering, or whatever you ultimately choose, know that the goal of this book is also to help you know what can go *right*, so you never have to worry about it going *wrong*. Plastic surgery is not just a medical procedure—it's an art. Any surgeon can become technically proficient over time, after doing hundreds of the same operations. The best plastic surgeons, though, have an *eye*, one that is as inimitable as Michelangelo's. They have the aesthetics. They have the instinctive skill to create a visual harmony in every face they work on, whether they're doing an easy chin implant or a complicated neck lift.

Plastic surgery is also, in a way, a *collaborative* art. It is my job to clearly explain to anyone sitting in my office, as I have in this book, what any kind of noninvasive or surgical procedure can actually do—to elaborate on the pros and be forthright about the cons. You will never hear me talk a patient into something unsuitable, or tell them what I think they *should* look like, or compare them to a celebrity. I am the first to say no when young patients want something done that will actually make them look older (such as fillers in the cheeks), or when patients want something that is wholly unnecessary for their facial structure (such as chin implants done in conjunction with a rhinoplasty) or that is physically impossible (such as trying to look exactly as they did fifty years ago).

It is your job to be honest about your expectations and why, precisely, you want to have a cosmetic procedure. I can't do that for you; your loved ones can't either. Suffice to say that there are many excellent reasons for wanting to have something done, and it is always a joy for me when a new patient comes to me prepared, is wholly forthcoming about these reasons, looks carefully at before-and-after photos, explicitly communicates what he or she wants, and listens to and follows all instructions to the letter. That is my ideal collaborator.

I think you know by now how much I love my job. Not only do I love the technical challenges that performing surgery entails—whether it's a very simple blepharoplasty or a very difficult revision on a botched nose job—but I love making my patients happy. I love listening to them tell me about themselves, and I love seeing their faces when they realize how wonderful they look afterward.

For now, I hope you will take the very best of the West Coast and East Coast styles and make it your own. Maybe, if you want larger lips, you'll go West Coast and ask for them to be a little larger than you originally considered, and you'll be stunned at how fabulous they look. Maybe, if you want more sculpted cheeks, you'll go East Coast and have custom implants made so they're perfection for your face. Whatever you decide, I wish you the best on your journey to actualizing the face you have dreamed of and envisioned!

Acknowledgments

I am grateful to have so many people who were instrumental in my development as a plastic surgeon, and I have many people to thank. It begins with my parents, who helped me realize that I had the ability to achieve my goals so long as I had the right work ethic. My grandfather Angelo Jacono, a master tailor, gave me the genetic ability to perform fine, precise work with my hands. My grandma Rose Jacono's kindness and concern for others inspired me to become a physician and later to perform pro bono plastic surgery on children with facial birth defects all over the world.

To my grade school classmate who was born with a cleft lip and palate deformity: Watching her transformation through plastic surgery confirmed my career path at a young age. It also made me passionate about my life's work to help restore facial harmony and balance and my patients' self-confidence.

I would not have developed my ability as a surgeon without my mentor, Vito Quatela, MD, who taught me how to perform the most complex reconstructive and cosmetic facial surgeries. I am grateful to all the American Academy of Facial Plastic and Reconstructive Surgery Fellows I have trained over the past decade, whose questions and curiosity helped me develop new techniques. To the countless colleagues all over the world whom I have lectured and listened to in conferences, you helped me evolve to deliver better care and outcomes to my patients.

I am thankful for my loyal nursing and professional staff who have helped me deliver the best care to my patients for almost twenty years: Georgette Deandressi, Harriet Feldman, Diane Spira, Joyce Mora, Luz Hidalgo, Joanne Mastroianni, Julie Stoller, Jamie Hands, Kelly Sheehan, Susie Maron, Laurie Slominski, Jacklyn Politi, and William Koontz. Their dedication and hard work can never be acknowledged enough on a day-to-day basis, and I do not know what I would do without them.

And, finally, to my patients, who have entrusted their faces to me: You have each brought joy into my life, and I feel like you are all members of my extended family.

Index

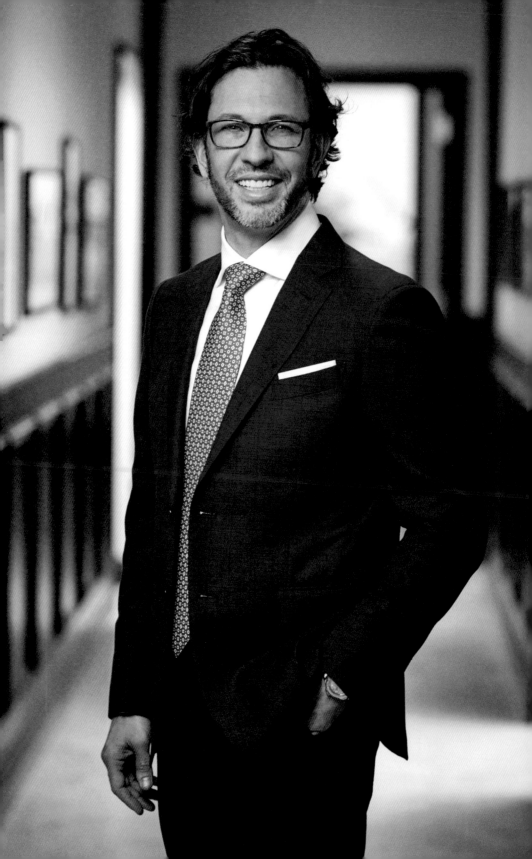

About the Author

Andrew Jacono, MD, FACS, is a global authority in the field of facial plastic and reconstructive surgery and is often called upon by colleagues and media around the world to provide his expert opinion. As one of New York City's premier plastic surgeons, Dr. Jacono is known for his original, advanced approach to nonsurgical and minimally invasive facial rejuvenation with flawless yet natural-appearing results. His current patient base consists of prominent American and international socialites, television news personalities, editors, models, and actors, as well as "everyday" women and men interested in rejuvenating their appearances.

Dr. Jacono is dual board certified (facial plastic and reconstructive surgery and head and neck surgery) and currently serves as Section Head of Facial Plastic and Reconstructive Surgery at North Shore University Hospital Manhasset, and as Associate Clinical Professor, Division of Facial Plastic and Reconstructive Surgery, at Albert Einstein College of Medicine. Additionally, Dr. Jacono serves as director of The New York Center for Facial Plastic and Laser Surgery in New York City, and as fellowship director of the American Academy of Facial Plastic and Reconstructive Surgery. He is not affiliated with any third-party, for-profit companies or organizations, making him an unbiased resource.

A Castle Connolly Top Doctor, Dr. Jacono has also been selected as one of America's Top Plastic Surgeons by the

Consumers' Research Council of America and Super Doctors. He was selected as one of the best facial plastic surgeons in New York City by *New York Magazine* and as one of the best plastic surgeons in America by *Harper's Bazaar*. He has also appeared on *Good Morning America, Anderson*, CNBC, and CNN, and in *USA Today, Town & Country, Departures, HuffPost, Esquire, Parade, O, The Oprah Magazine, Marie Claire*, and *GQ*, among others.

Dr. Jacono has presented clinical research and conducted live surgery in front of peer audiences at more than 100 plastic surgery meetings and symposiums around the world, hosted by International Master Course on Aging Skin (IMCAS), European Academy of Facial Plastic Surgery (EAFPS), International Society of Aesthetic Plastic Surgery (ISAPS), and American Academy of Facial Plastic and Reconstructive Surgery (AAFPRS), among others. He has delivered lectures on his innovative facelifting, eyelid lifting, and rhinoplasty techniques at the most prestigious universities in America, including Harvard University, Yale University, Stanford University, Columbia University, and the University of Pennsylvania. He has also published extensively in medical literature, with more than fifty articles appearing in peer-reviewed journals, including *Aesthetic Surgery Journal, JAMA Facial Plastic Surgery*, and *Aesthetic Plastic Surgery*.

In addition to his aesthetic work, Dr. Jacono volunteers for numerous charity organizations aimed at helping children throughout the world with limited medical and financial resources receive surgeries, including cleft lip and palate reconstruction. To date, Dr. Jacono has completed surgery on more than 500 children through missions with Healing the Children, the HUGS Foundation, and THAI Children, among others. He also serves as senior advisor to FACE TO FACE, a national project offering pro bono consultation and surgery to victims of domestic violence who have suffered facial disfigurement. To date, Dr. Jacono has provided pro bono reconstructive surgery to more than 100 female victims. His work with domestic violence victims was chronicled in the television series *Facing Trauma* on OWN and Discovery Fit & Health.